Osteochondritis Dissecans: Diagnosis and Treatment Options for Athletes

Editors

MATTHEW D. MILEWSKI
CARL W. NISSEN

CLINICS IN
SPORTS MEDICINE

www.sportsmed.theclinics.com

Consulting Editor
MARK D. MILLER

April 2014 • Volume 33 • Number 2

ELSEVIER

1600 John F. Kennedy Boulevard • Suite 1800 • Philadelphia, Pennsylvania, 19103-2899

http://www.theclinics.com

CLINICS IN SPORTS MEDICINE Volume 33, Number 2
April 2014 ISSN 0278-5919, ISBN-13: 978-0-323-29014-2

Editor: Jennifer Flynn-Briggs
Developmental Editor: Donald Mumford

Clinics in Sports Medicine (ISSN 0278-5919) is published quarterly by Elsevier Inc., 360 Park Avenue South, New York, NY 10010-1710. Months of issue are January, April, July, and October. Business and Editorial Offices: 1600 John F. Kennedy Blvd., Ste. 1800, Philadelphia, PA 19103-2899. Customer Service Office: 3251 Riverport Lane, Maryland Heights, MO 63043. Periodicals postage paid at New York, NY and additional mailing offices. Subscription prices are $340.00 per year (US individuals), $540.00 per year (US institutions), $165.00 per year (US students), $385.00 per year (Canadian individuals), $666.00 per year (Canadian institutions), $235.00 (Canadian students), $470.00 per year (foreign individuals), $666.00 per year (foreign institutions), and $235.00 per year (foreign students). Foreign air speed delivery is included in all *Clinics* subscription prices. All prices are subject to change without notice. **POSTMASTER:** Send address changes to *Clinics in Sports Medicine*, Elsevier Health Sciences Division, Subscription Customer Service, 3251 Riverport Lane, Maryland Heights, MO 63043. Customer Service (orders, claims, online, change of address): Elsevier Health Sciences Division, Subscription Customer Service, 3251 Riverport Lane, Maryland Heights, MO 63043. Tel: 1-800-654-2452 (U.S. and Canada); 314-447-8871 (outside U.S. and Canada). Fax: 314-447-8029. E-mail: journalscustomerservice-usa@elsevier.com (for print support); journalsonlinesupport-usa@elsevier.com (for online support).

Reprints. For copies of 100 or more of articles in this publication, please contact the Commercial Reprints Department, Elsevier Inc., 360 Park Avenue South, New York, NY 10010-1710. Tel.: 212-633-3874; Fax: 212-633-3820; E-mail: reprints@elsevier.com.

Clinics in Sports Medicine is covered in *MEDLINE/PubMed (Index Medicus) Current Contents/Clinical Medicine, Excerpta Medica,* and *ISI/Biomed.*

Printed and bound by CPI Group (UK) Ltd, Croydon, CR0 4YY

Contributors

CONSULTING EDITOR

MARK D. MILLER, MD
S. Ward Casscells Professor of Orthopaedic Surgery, University of Virginia; Team
Physician, James Madison University, JBJS Deputy Editor for Sports Medicine; Director,
Miller Review Course, Charlottesville, Virginia

EDITORS

MATTHEW D. MILEWSKI, MD
Elite Sports Medicine, Connecticut Children's Medical Center; Assistant Professor,
Department of Orthopaedic Surgery, University of Connecticut School of Medicine,
Farmington, Connecticut

CARL W. NISSEN, MD
Elite Sports Medicine, Connecticut Children's Medical Center; Professor, Department of
Orthopaedic Surgery, University of Connecticut School of Medicine, Farmington,
Connecticut

AUTHORS

JAY ALBRIGHT, MD
Children's Hospital Colorado, Aurora, Colorado

STEPHEN K. AOKI, MD
Department of Orthopaedics, University of Utah School of Medicine, Salt Lake City, Utah

NOAH ARCHIBALD-SEIFFER, BS
St. Luke's Health System, Boise, Idaho

J. TYLER BATES
Department of Biological Sciences, Biomolecular Research Center, Musculoskeletal
Research Institute, Boise State University, Boise, Idaho

LJILJANA BOGUNOVIC, MD
Department of Orthopedics, Washington University, St Louis, Missouri

JAMES L. CAREY, MD, MPH
Director of the Penn Center for Advanced Cartilage Repair and Osteochondritis Dissecans
Treatment, Assistant Professor of Orthopaedic Surgery, Perelman School of Medicine,
University of Pennsylvania, Philadelphia, Pennsylvania

ERIC W. EDMONDS, MD
Director of Orthopedic Research, Division of Orthopedic Surgery, Rady Children's
Hospital and Health Center; Assistant Professor, Department of Orthopedic Surgery,
University of California San Diego, San Diego, California

CHRISTOPHER K. EWING, DO
Department of Orthopaedics, Navy Medical Center San Diego, San Diego, California

THEODORE J. GANLEY, MD
Department of Orthopaedics, Sports Medicine and Performance Center, The Children's Hospital of Philadelphia, Philadelphia, Pennsylvania

NATHAN L. GRIMM, BS
Department of Orthopaedic Surgery, Duke University Medical Center, Durham, North Carolina

BENTON E. HEYWORTH, MD
Clinical Instructor in Orthopedic Surgery, Division of Sports Medicine, Department of Orthopedic Surgery, Boston Children's Hospital, Harvard Medical School, Boston, Massachusetts

JOHN C. JACOBS Jr, BS
University of Utah School of Medicine, Salt Lake City, Utah

JEFFREY I. KESSLER, MD
Department of Orthopaedics, Kaiser-Permanente Los Angeles, Los Angeles, California

MININDER S. KOCHER, MD
Associate Chief, Division of Sports Medicine, Professor of Orthopedic Surgery, Department of Orthopedic Surgery, Boston Children's Hospital, Harvard Medical School, Boston, Massachusetts

TAL LAOR, MD
Professor of Clinical Radiology, Department of Radiology, Cincinnati Children's Hospital Medical Center, University of Cincinnati College of Medicine, Cincinnati, Ohio

XUE-CHENG LIU, MD, PhD
Professor, Department of Orthopaedic Surgery, Children's Hospital of Wisconsin, Medical College of Wisconsin, Milwaukee, Wisconsin

ROGER LYON, MD
Professor, Department of Orthopaedic Surgery, Children's Hospital of Wisconsin, Medical College of Wisconsin, Milwaukee, Wisconsin

MATTHEW D. MILEWSKI, MD
Elite Sports Medicine, Connecticut Children's Medical Center; Assistant Professor, Department of Orthopaedic Surgery, University of Connecticut School of Medicine, Farmington, Connecticut

M. LUCAS MURNAGHAN, MD, MEd, FRCSC
Assistant Professor, Department of Surgery, University of Toronto; Division of Orthopaedics, The Hospital for Sick Children, Toronto, Ontario, Canada

CARL W. NISSEN, MD
Elite Sports Medicine, Connecticut Children's Medical Center; Professor, Department of Orthopaedic Surgery, University of Connecticut School of Medicine, Farmington, Connecticut

JULIA THOM OXFORD, PhD
Department of Biological Sciences, Biomolecular Research Center, Musculoskeletal Research Institute, Boise State University, Boise, Idaho

MARK V. PATERNO, PT, PhD, SCS, ATC
Cincinnati Children's Hospital Medical Center; Division of Occupational Therapy and Physical Therapy; Division of Sports Medicine; Department of Pediatrics, College of Medicine, University of Cincinnati, Cincinnati, Ohio

JOHN D. POLOUSKY, MD
Surgical Director-Sports Medicine, The Rocky Mountain Youth Sports Medicine Institute, Centennial, Colorado

TRICIA R. PROKOP, PT, MS, CSCS
Physical Therapist, Connecticut Children's Medical Center, Department of Physical Therapy, Division of Sports Medicine; Part-Time Faculty, Department of Rehabilitation Sciences, College of Education, Nursing, and Health Professions, University of Hartford, West Hartford, Connecticut

LAURA C. SCHMITT, PT, PhD
Assistant Professor, Division of Physical Therapy, School of Health and Rehabilitation Sciences, Ohio State University, Columbus; Cincinnati Children's Hospital Medical Center; Division of Sports Medicine, Cincinnati, Ohio

KEVIN G. SHEA, MD
Orthopedic Surgeon, St. Luke's Sports Medicine, St. Luke's Health System, St. Luke's Children's Hospital, Boise, Idaho; Adjunct Associate Clinical Professor, Department of Orthopedics, University of Utah, Salt Lake City, Utah

PAUL G. TALUSAN, MD
Orthopaedic Surgery Resident, Department of Orthopaedics & Rehabilitation, Yale University School of Medicine, New Haven, Connecticut

JASON O. TOY, MD
Orthopaedic Surgery Resident, Department of Orthopaedics & Rehabilitation, Yale University School of Medicine, New Haven, Connecticut

ERIC J. WALL, MD
Professor, Department of Surgery, University of Cincinnati School of Medicine; Division of Orthopaedic Surgery, Cincinnati Children's Hospital Medical Center, Cincinnati, Ohio

JENNIFER M. WEISS, MD
Department of Orthopaedics, Kaiser-Permanente Los Angeles, Los Angeles, California

RICK W. WRIGHT, MD
Department of Orthopedics, Washington University, St Louis, Missouri

JUSTIN S. YANG, MD
Department of Orthopedics, Washington University, St Louis, Missouri

ANDREW M. ZBOJNIEWICZ, MD
Assistant Professor of Clinical Radiology, Department of Radiology, Cincinnati Children's Hospital Medical Center, University of Cincinnati College of Medicine, Cincinnati, Ohio

Contents

Although several hypotheses have been described to explain the cause
of osteochondritis dissecans, no single hypothesis has been accepted in
the orthopedic community. Given its increased incidence among athletes, most in the sports medicine community agree that repetitive
microtrauma plays at least some role in its development. Knowledge
regarding the epidemiology and pathoanatomy of osteochondritis dissecans has helped the understanding of osteochondritis dissecans; however, much is still to be learned about this condition and its cause.
This article reviews the history of osteochondritis as it pertains to the
current understanding of its pathoanatomy, epidemiology, and diagnostic features.

Multiple systems for classifying osteochondritis dissecans (OCD) of the
knee have been reported. These existing classification systems have
some similar characteristics, such as stable lesion/intact articular cartilage
and presence of a loose body. However, variations are found in the number of stages and specific lesion characteristics assessed. Currently, no
system has been universally accepted. A future classification system
should be developed that reconciles the discrepancies among the current
systems and provides a clear, consistent, and reliable method for classifying OCD lesions of the knee during arthroscopy.

Genome-wide association studies (GWAS) provide an unbiased approach
in the identification of genes that increase the risk for osteochondritis dissecans (OCD). Recent GWAS in humans, horses, and pigs are reviewed
and genes identified. The identified genes tended to cluster with respect
to function and biologic processes. GWAS in humans are a critical next
step in the effort to provide a better understanding of the causes of
OCD, which will, in turn, allow preventive strategies for treatment of adolescents and young adults who are at risk for the development of degenerative joint disease due to the effects of OCD.

Osteochondritis dissecans (OCD) can affect both adults and children, however the imaging characteristics and significance of imaging findings can differ in the juvenile subset with open physes. Radiography and magnetic resonance imaging (MRI) are the primary modalities used to aid in diagnosis, to define a treatment plan, to monitor progress, to assess surgical intervention, and to identify postoperative complications. Newer imaging techniques under continuous development may improve the accuracy of MRI for diagnosis and staging of OCD, and eventually may help to predict the durability of tissue-engineered constructs and cartilage repair.

Osteochondritis dissecans affects the elbow of many young, skeletally immature athletes. The incidence of OCD in the elbow is second to its occurrence in the knee and similar to the incidence in the ankle. Young, athletically active individuals are at increased risk for developing this problem. There is a predilection for those involved in overhead-dominant sports and sports that require the arm to be a weight-bearing limb. The diagnosis is occurring earlier because of an increased awareness of the entity and the increased use of advanced imaging techniques, primarily magnetic resonance imaging. This earlier diagnosis has led to an increase in treatment ideas and modalities and ultimately improved care and outcomes.

Osteochondritis dissecans of the talus is a subset of osteochondral lesions of the talus that also includes osteochondral fractures, avascular necrosis, and degenerative arthritis. Osteochondral lesions of the talus can be associated with injury to the ankle. This article discusses the anatomy, pathoanatomy, history, physical examination, imaging, management algorithm, and outcomes of surgical treatment of osteochondral lesions in these patients. This article also presents the authors' recommended surgical technique.

Shoulder and hip osteochondritis dissecans (OCD) are uncommon. Both glenoid and humeral head OCD are commonly associated with a traumatic etiology. Humeral head OCD can be treated with observation or drilling of the sclerotic margin for stable or unstable lesions. Glenoid OCD often presents with delamination of the articular cartilage and requires debridement and fixation of fragments. Hip OCD often involves the femoral head; yet, there are case reports of acetabular involvement. The etiology of femoral OCD is associated with other pathologies, and therefore may represent the sequelae of other disease processes. Hip lesions often require extensive surgical intervention.

CLINICS IN SPORTS MEDICINE

FORTHCOMING ISSUES

July 2014
Understanding the Patellofemoral Joint:
From Instability to Arthroplasty
Alex Meininger, MD, *Editor*

October 2014
Sports Injuries in the Military
Brett D. Owens, MD, *Editor*

RECENT ISSUES

January 2014
Unicompartmental Knee Arthroplasty
Kevin D. Plancher, MD and
Stephanie C. Petterson PhD, *Editors*

October 2013
Shoulder Instability in the Athlete
Stephen Thompson, MD, *Editor*

July 2013
Blunt MRI in Sports Medicine
Timothy G. Sanders, *Editor*

April 2013
Blunt Trauma Injuries in the Athlete
Thomas M. DeBerardino, MD, *Editor*

RELATED INTEREST

Orthopedic Clinics of North America, January 2014 (Vol. 45, No. 1)
http://www.orthopedic.theclinics.com/current

NOW AVAILABLE FOR YOUR iPhone and iPad

Preface

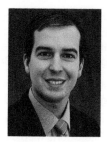
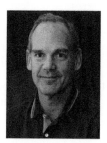

Matthew D. Milewski, MD   Carl W. Nissen, MD
Editors

We have been privileged to serve as editors for this issue of *Clinics in Sports Medicine* dedicated to Osteochondritis Dissecans (OCD). Since König[1] first coined the term in 1887, this unique disease process has challenged health care providers as to its true etiology and treatment. A recent Clinical Practice Guidelines[2] (CPG) sponsored by the American Academy of Orthopaedics Surgeons (AAOS) and put together by leading experts highlighted the lack of high-quality evidence-based definitive diagnostic and treatment recommendations. However, spurred by these findings, a group of international surgeons, musculoskeletal radiologists, physical therapists, and researchers formed the Research in Osteochondritis of the Knee (ROCK) group[3] to try and answer these questions. Many of the articles are written by members of this prestigious group, who provide their vast experience and knowledge on the subject.

The issue focuses on OCD, defined herein as "a focal, idiopathic alteration of subchondral bone with risk for instability and disruption of adjacent articular cartilage that may result in premature osteoarthritis"[4] with particular attention to student-athletes. The invited authors clearly shed light on the pathophysiology, possible etiologies, including genetic predisposition, imaging characteristics, unique rehabilitation strategies, and treatment options ranging from nonoperative conservative strategies to salvage procedures, and even future cutting-edge options. While much of the focus in this issue centers on OCD of the knee, individual articles are also dedicated to OCD of the elbow, talus, shoulder, and hip.

We hope that this issue serves the reader in shedding light on this unique disease process to improve provider and patient education, understand the various treatment strategies and possible outcomes, and spur further interest in researching this disease

Clin Sports Med 33 (2014) xiii–xiv
http://dx.doi.org/10.1016/j.csm.2014.01.005
0278-5919/14/$ – see front matter © 2014 Published by Elsevier Inc.

sportsmed.theclinics.com

process to improve the care of athletes and all patients and families affected by Osteochondritis Dissecans.

Matthew D. Milewski, MD
Elite Sports Medicine
Connecticut Children's Medical Center
Farmington, CT 06032, USA

University of Connecticut School of Medicine
Farmington, CT 06030, USA

Carl W. Nissen, MD
Elite Sports Medicine
Connecticut Children's Medical Center
Farmington, CT 06032, USA

University of Connecticut School of Medicine
Farmington, CT 06030, USA

E-mail addresses:
mdmilewski@gmail.com (M.D. Milewski)
cnissen@ccmckids.org (C.W. Nissen)

REFERENCES

1. König F. Ueber freie Körper in den Gelenken. [On loose bodies in the joint]. Dtsch Z Chir 1887;27:90–109.
2. Chambers HG, Shea KG, Carey JL. AAOS Clinical Practice Guideline: diagnosis and treatment of osteochondritis dissecans. J Am Acad Orthop Surg 2011;19: 307–9.
3. Research in Osteochondritis Dissecans of the Knee (ROCK) Group. Available at: http://www.osteochondritisdissecans.org and http://www.kneeocd.org. Accessed January 3, 2014.
4. Edmonds EW, Shea KG. Osteochondritis dissecans. Editorial comment. Clin Orthop Relat Res 2013;471:1105–6.

Osteochondritis Dissecans of the Knee

Pathoanatomy, Epidemiology, and Diagnosis

Nathan L. Grimm, BS[a,b,*], Jennifer M. Weiss, MD[c],
Jeffrey I. Kessler, MD[c], Stephen K. Aoki, MD[d]

KEYWORDS

- Osteochondritis dissecans • Osteochondrosis • Sports medicine • Knee
- Epidemiology

KEY POINTS

- Multiple hypotheses exist regarding the cause of osteochondritis dissecans (OCD); leading theories at this point are those of repetitive microtrauma, disruption of normal endochondral ossification, and genetic factors.
- Male/female ratio is approximately 4:1 and the highest incidence in the United States is seen in the African American population.
- Plain radiographs, especially the flexion notch view, are important in the diagnosis of OCD lesions, whereas magnetic resonance imaging is paramount for OCD lesion characterization.
- Arthroscopy continues to be the gold standard for assessing the stability of OCD lesions.

INTRODUCTION

It has been more than 125 years since German-born, Franz König[1] first described and coined the term osteochondritis dissecans (OCD).[1,2] Since its early characterization, OCD has remained enigmatic and the evolution of its understanding has been slow in the orthopedic community. Confusion about the pathoanatomy and cause of OCD is partially derived from the roots of its etymology. The suffix -itis in

There was no outside funding for this study.
The authors have nothing to disclose.
[a] Department of Orthopaedics, Intermountain Orthopaedics, 600 Robbins Road, Boise, ID 83702, USA; [b] Department of Orthopaedics, University of Utah School of Medicine, 1311 Medical Plaza, Salt Lake City, UT 84112, USA; [c] Department of Orthopaedics, Kaiser-Permanente Los Angeles, 4760 Sunset Boulevard, Los Angeles, CA 90027, USA; [d] Department of Orthopaedics, University of Utah School of Medicine, 590 Wakara Way, Salt Lake City, UT 84103, USA
* Corresponding author. Department of Orthopaedics, University of Utah School of Medicine, 1311 Medical Plaza, Salt Lake City, UT 84112.
E-mail address: nathan.grimm@hsc.utah.edu

osteochondritis comes from the Greek root meaning inflammation, despite the current belief that inflammation plays little to no role in the pathoanatomy of OCD. In an attempt to standardize language for discussing OCD lesions, the Research in Osteochondritis Dissecans of the Knee (ROCK) group[3] has defined the term OCD as a focal, idiopathic alteration of subchondral bone with risk for instability and disruption of adjacent articular cartilage that may result in premature osteoarthritis.[4]

Researchers have proposed several hypotheses for the causes of OCD, which have included occult or repetitive microtrauma,[5–8] genetic predisposition and markers,[9–12] inflammatory causation,[1,13] and vascular abnormalities.[14,15] However, despite these hypotheses, there has been no conclusive agreement on the cause. Nonetheless, given its increased incidence in people participating in athletics, a repetitive microtrauma hypothesis is the most popular and can also account for the increased incidence of medial femoral condyle lesions of the knee given the location's proximity to the tibial eminence. However, this hypothesis cannot explain the causal development of OCD in other locations and joints.

Classification of OCD in the knee is broken down by lesion location, characterization of the lesion, status of the overlying cartilage, and skeletal maturity. These variables are elucidated with the use of radiographs, magnetic resonance imaging (MRI), and direct visualization through arthroscopy and/or open arthrotomy in certain cases.

This article provides a detailed review of OCD of the knee, with specific discussions on pathoanatomy, epidemiology, and the diagnosis of OCD.

CAUSES OF OCD
Inflammatory Causes

As previously mentioned, the hypotheses include inflammatory, vascular, trauma/microtrauma, and genetic causes. OCD was first thought by König[1] to have an inflammatory component, hence the suffix itis. Despite describing what König[1] described as "dissecting inflammation," early histologic analysis of loose bodies in OCD suggested that an inflammatory component is unlikely.[16,17]

Vascular/Ischemic Causes

Eighteen years before König[1] coined the term OCD, Sir James Paget[18] described what was later thought to be OCD as "quiet necrosis." In the same vein, Green and Banks[19] also theorized that OCD was caused by ischemia/necrosis of subchondral bone leading to the development of OCD. Researchers in the early twentieth century had several hypotheses for the cause of these ischemic/vascular insults. These hypotheses included emboli from tubercle bacilli,[20] fat emboli,[21] and blood emboli.[22] However, the crux of the hypotheses relied on the supposition that the epiphyseal arterial supply was an end artery construct, which was later shown not to be the case. Moreover, histopathologic analysis of excised OCD specimens has suggested that avascular necrosis is not the cause.[23]

Trauma/Microtrauma

Although both Paget and König discussed trauma in their early works, it was Fairbanks[24] in the early twentieth century who championed the hypothesis of trauma as a cause for OCD. Despite the inability to explain OCD in other joints without clear impaction-type injuries, Smillie[8] strongly supported Fairbanks's[24] so-called tibial spine theory for the cause of OCD. In addition, the work of Cahill[25–27] and Cahill and Berg[28] suggests that earlier sport entry results in juvenile OCD occurring in the weight-bearing portions of the femoral condyle. Perhaps a theory of repetitive microtrauma is appealing given that multiple studies have shown that up to 60% of patients with OCD report being involved in sporting activities.[29–31] Nonetheless, this theory, like many others, has gaps that cannot be accounted for.

Hereditary/Genetic Causes

A solitary lesion located in the lateral aspect of the medial femoral condyle is the most commonly reported OCD in the literature. However, episodes of joint bilaterality,[6,32] multiple lesions in a single joint,[33,34] and reports of OCD in twin studies[35,36] have provided support for a hypotheses of genetic predisposition. Studies have suggested a possible mendelian inheritance pattern seen with OCD.[10,11,37] Furthermore, Swedish researchers have identified the *ACAN* gene, which is important for cartilage function, as a cause for dominant familial OCD.[38] Although this is a step toward providing an explanation for the molecular mechanism of OCD, larger pedigree analyses are needed to determine a discrete inheritance pattern.

Endochondral Ossification/Secondary Centers of Ossification

As pointed out by Edmonds and Polousky,[39] the only hypothesis that may unite all previous evidence is that of epiphyseal endochondral ossification, which was described by Ribbing.[40] These accessory centers of ossification were championed by Ribbing[40] and shown to occur in the classic location of the medial femoral condyle. More convincingly, in Ribbing's[40] 1955 article he provides an eloquently described explanation and anecdote for how an accessory center of ossification can function as a locus minoris resistentiae (nidus) to develop into what is now known as an OCD lesion.[40] Combining nearly all theories into one, Ribbing[40] reports:

> The etiology of osteochondritis dissecans is complex; it is both constitutional and traumatic. An accessory bone nucleus, detached in childhood, during adolescence partly fuses into the adjacent cancellous bone and strands of persisting cartilage. There is incomplete collateral connection between the vascular system of the bone nucleus and that of the vicinity. This bone nucleus constitutes the locus minoris resistentiae [nidus] which enables mild injury or strain – perhaps even within the range of normal function – to produce a slight dislocation with deleterious action upon the blood supply of the bone nucleus.

EPIDEMIOLOGY OF OCD

The first true epidemiologic analysis of knee OCD was performed over a 10-year period (1963–1974) by Bjarne Linden.[31] Using hospital data from the general hospital in Malmö, Sweden, Linden[31] quantified the incidence of OCD in patients less than 50 years of age. The data were extrapolated from patients diagnosed via radiographic means or operative findings. Linden[31] showed that the incidence for both women and men varied with age, and that the highest incidence for both occurred between the ages of 10 and 20 years, which was approximately 18 in 100,000 for women and 28 in 100,000 for men[31] in this age group. The ratio of incidence for men to women was nearly 2:1. In addition, there was a predilection for OCD lesions to occur in the lateral aspect of the medial femoral condyle; the so-called classic location. The distribution of the location of knee OCD findings was consistent with other estimations based on smaller samples.[29,41]

Kessler and colleagues and members of the ROCK group recently collected data from a cohort of more than 1 million individuals aged from 2 to 19 years that have yielded similar distributions of knee OCD (Kessler JI, Hooman N, Shea KG, et al, unpublished data, 2013). However, Kessler's study showed an even greater risk for men

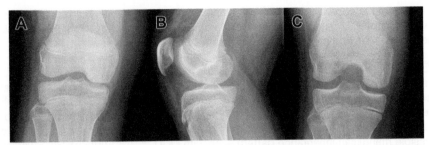

Fig. 1. Anterior-posterior (*A*), lateral (*B*), and notch views (*C*). Note that the lesion is best appreciated on the notch view.

versus women than that of Linden,[31] with an overall ratio of approximately 4:1. Furthermore, when stratified by race, this study showed that African Americans had the highest odds ratio of knee OCD (Kessler JI, Hooman N, Shea KG, et al, unpublished data, 2013).

DIAGNOSIS OF OCD

The diagnosis of OCD is based on a multifaceted approach beginning with a thorough history and physical examination and then further characterization with plain radiographs and MRI. Specific physical examination tests such as the Wilson[42] sign are unreliable and nonspecific.[43] There is anecdotal evidence that patients presenting with an OCD lesion may present in a variety of ways including with activity-related pain, catching or locking of the affected joint, and/or a transient effusion. The painful symptoms may mimic patellofemoral disorders. The physical examiner should pay special attention to body habitus, biomechanical subtleties in gait, location of tenderness/ pain, and alleviating and aggravating factors.

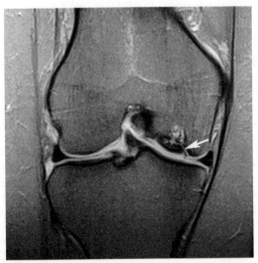

Fig. 2. OCD lesion of the knee with distinct fragment and line of high signal intensity (*white arrow*) between the progeny and parent bone.

Radiographs are useful for making the diagnosis of OCD. Of key importance in identifying potential OCD lesions are the lateral[44,45] and notch[45] views for appreciating the location of the lesion (**Fig. 1**). Although some investigators describe poor reliability with radiographs,[46–48] Mesgarzadeh and colleagues[49] reported that plain radiographs are indispensable in the initial detection of OCD lesions.

The usefulness of MRI for diagnosing soft tissue and chondral defects is well established; MRI use in diagnosing and further characterizing OCD lesions is paramount. Several studies' classification systems[48,50,51] for characterizing knee OCD lesions are based on MRI findings. These classifications uniformly agree that the following signs reliably indicate the stability, or instability, of OCD lesions: distinct fragments, high T-2 signal intensity between the parent and progeny bone, chondral disruption, and identifiable loose bodies (**Fig. 2**). The sensitivity and specificity of MRI has been reported to be as high as 92% to 100%,[47,49,52,53] respectively. However, despite the impressive sensitivity and specificity of this imaging modality, arthroscopy continues to be the gold or reference standard for diagnosing stability.[54]

SUMMARY

Despite more than 125 years of recognition, the exact cause of OCD has yet to be elucidated in humans. Bolder statements in the veterinary medical community have been made, such as that "...the veterinary field is far ahead of the human field with respect to the unambiguous definition of [OCD] as a failure of the process of endochondral ossification of the epiphyseal articular complex."[55] Perhaps their understanding comes from their greater ability to study a disease that is more common in animals, with a prevalence as high as 67% in animal patients.[56,57] This percentage contrasts with the approximate 9 in 100,000 incidence seen in their human counterparts (Kessler JI, Hooman N, Shea KG, et al, unpublished data, 2013).

As Edmonds and Polousky[39] point out, OCD is a rare condition, making it difficult for any single surgeon to treat enough cases to perform any meaningful comparative research. This difficulty is shown by the small number of articles identified by the American Academy of Orthopaedic Surgeons Clinical Practice Guidelines Committee as making recommendations on the diagnosis and treatment of OCD.[54] Nonetheless, with the development of research groups such as the ROCK group,[3] it is likely that future high-quality, prospective, comparative research will provide a better understanding of the cause, diagnosis, and treatment of OCD lesions.

REFERENCES

1. König F. Uber freie Körper in den Gelenken. Dtsch Z Klin Chir 1887;27:90–109.
2. Brand RA. Biographical sketch: Franz Konig, MD 1832–1910. Clin Orthop Relat Res 2013;471(4):1116–7.
3. Research in osteochondritis dissecans of the knee (ROCK). 2013. Available at: http://kneeocd.org. Accessed 20 August, 2013.
4. Edmonds EW, Shea KG. Osteochondritis dissecans: editorial comment. Clin Orthop Relat Res 2013;471(4):1105–6.
5. Conway FM. Osteochondritis dissecans. Description of the stages of the condition and its probable traumatic etiology. Am J Surg 1937;38(3):691–9.
6. Crawford DC, Safran MR. Osteochondritis dissecans of the knee. J Am Acad Orthop Surg 2006;14(2):90–100.
7. Detterline AJ, Goldstein JL, Rue JP, et al. Evaluation and treatment of osteochondritis dissecans lesions of the knee. J Knee Surg 2008;21(2):106–15.

8. Smillie IS. Treatment of osteochondritis dissecans. J Bone Joint Surg Br 1957; 39(2):248–60.

9. Andrew TA, Spivey J, Lindebaum RH. Familial osteochondritis dissecans and dwarfism. Acta Orthop Scand 1981;52(5):519–23.

10. Kozlowski K, Middleton R. Familial osteochondritis dissecans: a dysplasia of articular cartilage? Skeletal Radiol 1985;13(3):207–10.

11. Phillips HO, Grubb SA. Familial multiple osteochondritis dissecans. Report of a kindred. J Bone Joint Surg Am 1985;67(1):155–6.

12. Stougaard J. Familial occurrence of osteochondritis dissecans. J Bone Joint Surg Br 1964;46:542–3.

13. Schenck RC Jr, Goodnight JM. Osteochondritis dissecans. J Bone Joint Surg Am 1996;78(3):439–56.

14. Campbell CJ, Ranawat CS. Osteochondritis dissecans: the question of etiology. J Trauma 1966;6(2):201–21.

15. Linden B, Telhag H. Osteochondritis dissecans. A histologic and autoradiographic study in man. Acta Orthop Scand 1977;48(6):682–6.

16. Barrie HJ. Hypertrophy and laminar calcification of cartilage in loose bodies as probable evidence of an ossification abnormality. J Pathol 1980;132(2):161–8.

17. Barrie HJ. Hypothesis–a diagram of the form and origin of loose bodies in osteochondritis dissecans. J Rheumatol 1984;11(4):512–3.

18. Paget J. On the production of some of the loose bodies in joints. Saint Bartholomew's Hospital Reports 1870;6.

19. Green WT, Banks HH. Osteochondritis dissecans in children. J Bone Joint Surg Am 1953;35(1):26–47 passim.

20. Axhausen G. Die Aetiologie der Kohler'schen Erkrankung der Metatarsalkopfchen. Beitr Klin Chir 1922;(126):451.

21. Rieger H. Zur Pathogenese von Gelenkmausen. Munchener Medizinische Wochenschrift 1920;(67):719.

22. Watson-Jones SR, editor. Fractures and joint injuries, vol. 1, 4th edition. Edinburgh (United Kingdom), London: E & S Livingston; 1952.

23. Milgram JW. Radiological and pathological manifestations of osteochondritis dissecans of the distal femur. Radiology 1978;126(2):305–11.

24. Fairbanks H. Osteo-chondritis dissecans. Br J Surg 1933;21(81):67–82.

25. Cahill B. Treatment of juvenile osteochondritis dissecans and osteochondritis dissecans of the knee. Clin Sports Med 1985;4(2):367–84.

26. Cahill BR. Osteochondritis dissecans of the knee: treatment of juvenile and adult forms. J Am Acad Orthop Surg 1995;3(4):237–47.

27. Cahill BR. Current concepts review. Osteochondritis dissecans. J Bone Joint Surg Am 1997;79(3):471–2.

28. Cahill BR, Berg BC. 99m-Technetium phosphate compound joint scintigraphy in the management of juvenile osteochondritis dissecans of the femoral condyles. Am J Sports Med 1983;11(5):329–35.

29. Aichroth P. Osteochondritis dissecans of the knee. A clinical survey. J Bone Joint Surg Br 1971;53(3):440–7.

30. Hefti F, Beguiristain J, Krauspe R, et al. Osteochondritis dissecans: a multicenter study of the European Pediatric Orthopedic Society. J Pediatr Orthop B 1999; 8(4):231–45.

31. Linden B. The incidence of osteochondritis dissecans in the condyles of the femur. Acta Orthop Scand 1976;47(6):664–7.

32. Robertson W, Kelly BT, Green DW. Osteochondritis dissecans of the knee in children. Curr Opin Pediatr 2003;15(1):38–44.

33. Grimm NL, Tisano B, Carey JL. Three osteochondritis dissecans lesions in one knee: a case report. Clin Orthop Relat Res 2013;471(4):1186–90.

34. Hanna SA, Aston WJ, Gikas PD, et al. Bicondylar osteochondritis dissecans in the knee: a report of two cases. J Bone Joint Surg Br 2008;90(2):232–5.

35. Mackie T, Wilkins RM. Case report: osteochondritis dissecans in twins: treatment with fresh osteochondral grafts. Clin Orthop Relat Res 2010;468(3):893–7.

36. Mei-Dan O, Mann G, Steinbacher G, et al. Bilateral osteochondritis dissecans of the knees in monozygotic twins: the genetic factor and review of the etiology. Am J Orthop 2009;38(9):E152–5.

37. Mubarak SJ, Carroll NC. Familial osteochondritis dissecans of the knee. Clin Orthop Relat Res 1979;(140):131–6.

38. Stattin EL, Wiklund F, Lindblom K, et al. A missense mutation in the aggrecan C-type lectin domain disrupts extracellular matrix interactions and causes dominant familial osteochondritis dissecans. Am J Hum Genet 2010;86(2):126–37.

39. Edmonds EW, Polousky J. A review of knowledge in osteochondritis dissecans: 123 years of minimal evolution from Konig to the ROCK study group. Clin Orthop Relat Res 2013;471(4):1118–26.

40. Ribbing S. The hereditary multiple epiphyseal disturbance and its consequences for the aetiogenesis of local malacias–particularly the osteochondrosis dissecans. Acta Orthop Scand 1955;24(4):286–99.

41. Green JP. Osteochondritis dissecans of the knee. J Bone Joint Surg Br 1966; 48(1):82–91.

42. Wilson JN. A diagnostic sign in osteochondritis dissecans of the knee. J Bone Joint Surg Am 1967;49(3):477–80.

43. Conrad JM, Stanitski CL. Osteochondritis dissecans: Wilson's sign revisited. Am J Sports Med 2003;31(5):777–8.

44. Harding WG 3rd. Diagnosis of osteochondritis dissecans of the femoral condyles: the value of the lateral x-ray view. Clin Orthop Relat Res 1977;(123):25–6.

45. Kocher MS, Czarnecki JJ, Andersen JS, et al. Internal fixation of juvenile osteochondritis dissecans lesions of the knee. Am J Sports Med 2007;35(5):712–8.

46. Wall E, Von Stein D. Juvenile osteochondritis dissecans. Orthop Clin North Am 2003;34(3):341–53.

47. O'Connor MA, Palaniappan M, Khan N, et al. Osteochondritis dissecans of the knee in children. A comparison of MRI and arthroscopic findings. J Bone Joint Surg Br 2002;84(2):258–62.

48. Dipaola JD, Nelson DW, Colville MR. Characterizing osteochondral lesions by magnetic resonance imaging. Arthroscopy 1991;7(1):101–4.

49. Mesgarzadeh M, Sapega AA, Bonakdarpour A, et al. Osteochondritis dissecans: analysis of mechanical stability with radiography, scintigraphy, and MR imaging. Radiology 1987;165(3):775–80.

50. Bohndorf K. Osteochondritis (osteochondrosis) dissecans: a review and new MRI classification. Eur Radiol 1998;8(1):103–12.

51. Kramer J, Stiglbauer R, Engel A, et al. MR contrast arthrography (MRA) in osteochondrosis dissecans. J Comput Assist Tomogr 1992;16(2):254–60.

52. Samora WP, Chevillet J, Adler B, et al. Juvenile osteochondritis dissecans of the knee: predictors of lesion stability. J Pediatr Orthop 2012;32(1):1–4.

53. Kijowski R, Blankenbaker DG, Shinki K, et al. Juvenile versus adult osteochondritis dissecans of the knee: appropriate MR imaging criteria for instability. Radiology 2008;248(2):571–8.

54. Clinical practice guideline on the diagnosis and treatment of osteochondritis dissecans Rosemont (IL). Guideline and Evidence Report American Academy

of Orthopaedic Surgeons (AAOS). 1st edition. 2010. Available at: http://www.aaos.org/research/guidelines/guide.asp. Accessed 20 August, 2013.

55. van Weeren PR, Jeffcott LB. Problems and pointers in osteochondrosis: twenty years on. Vet J 2013;197(1):96–102.

56. Dik KJ, Enzerink E, van Weeren PR. Radiographic development of osteochondral abnormalities, in the hock and stifle of Dutch warmblood foals, from age 1 to 11 months. Equine Vet J Suppl 1999;(31):9–15.

57. van Grevenhof EM, Ducro BJ, van Weeren PR, et al. Prevalence of various radiographic manifestations of osteochondrosis and their correlations between and within joints in Dutch warmblood horses. Equine Vet J 2009;41(1):11–6.

A Review of Arthroscopic Classification Systems for Osteochondritis Dissecans of the Knee

John C. Jacobs Jr, BS[a],*, Noah Archibald-Seiffer, BS[b],
Nathan L. Grimm, BS[c], James L. Carey, MD, MPH[d],
Kevin G. Shea, MD[e]

KEYWORDS

- Osteochondritis dissecans • Arthroscopy • Knee • Classification • Grading
- Stability

KEY POINTS

- Multiple systems have been described for classifying osteochondritis dissecans (OCD) lesions of the knee during arthroscopy, with varying levels of overlap among the existing classification systems.
- The identified classification systems associate intact articular cartilage with lesion stability, whereas instability is associated with a disruption of the articular cartilage.
- None of the studies included in this review rigorously assessed the inter-rater and intra-rater reliability of an arthroscopic grading system for OCD lesions of the knee.
- Future research is needed to establish a classification system for OCD of the knee during arthroscopy that demonstrates high inter-rater and intra-rater reliability.

INTRODUCTION

Osteochondritis dissecans (OCD) is a focal, idiopathic alteration of subchondral bone with potential for instability and disruption of adjacent articular cartilage that may result in premature osteoarthritis.[1] Several risk factors have been linked to OCD of the knee,

Disclosures: None of the authors has any relationships with any commercial companies.
[a] University of Utah School of Medicine, 30 North 1900 East, Salt Lake City, UT 84132, USA;
[b] St. Luke's Health System, 1109 West Myrtle Road, Suite 220, Boise, ID 83702, USA;
[c] Department of Orthopaedic Surgery, Duke University Medical Center, Box 3956, Durham, NC 27710, USA; [d] Penn Center for Advanced Cartilage Repair and Osteochondritis Dissecans Treatment, Perelman School of Medicine, University of Pennsylvania, Weightman Hall, 1st floor, 235 South 33rd Street, Philadelphia, PA 19104, USA; [e] Department of Orthopedics, St. Luke's Sports Medicine, St. Luke's Children's Hospital, University of Utah, 600 West Robbins Road, Boise, ID 83702, USA
* Corresponding author.
E-mail address: jacobsjc013@gmail.com

including male sex, age (with 10–20 years being at highest risk), sports participation, and African-American ethnicity.[2–4] Three primary methods have been used to assess the stability, severity, and potential for healing of the OCD lesion: radiographs, magnetic resonance imaging (MRI), and arthroscopy. Although many methods have been developed to classify the various stages of OCD lesions, none has been rigorously validated for accuracy, ease of use, or prognostic predictive ability.

The main principle underlying the classification of OCD lesions focuses on the stability of the lesion. The term *stability*, in regard to OCD lesions, has been used to describe the mechanical integrity and stability of the subchondral OCD lesion.[5] Furthermore, characteristics of a stable lesion (**Figs. 1** and **2**) include those that have stable articular cartilage, whereas a disruption in the articular cartilage (**Fig. 3**) is present in lesions that are usually loose or unstable (**Fig. 4**).[5] Some lesions may be stable but do include a breech in the articular cartilage.[6]

Multiple grading systems exist for classifying OCD of the knee during arthroscopic surgery. However, variation among these classifications and the lack of a standardized method for grading OCD lesions prevents comparison among the published literature on arthroscopy of OCD of the knee. This article reviews the English-written literature for existing systems for classifying OCD lesions of the knee during arthroscopic surgery.

REVIEW OF THE LITERATURE
Radiographic and MRI Classifications

Berndt and Harty[7] described one of the first classification systems in 1959. They classified talar OCD lesions on radiographic images, with stages ranging from a small area of compression of the subchondral bone to a completely detached fragment or loose body. Rodegerdts and Gleissner[8,9] described an early classification system for OCD of the knee in 1981. They classified lesions on radiographic images, with 5 stages ranging from a potentially depressed osteochondral fracture to a displaced fragment or loose body. Subsequent authors have described additional radiographic methods of classification, all with various ranges of modifications and reclassifications.[5,7,10,11]

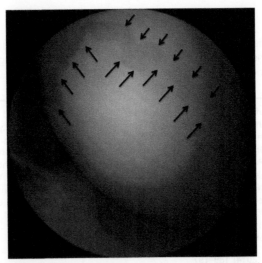

Fig. 1. Stable OCD lesion with clearly delineated border (*black arrows*). Lesion is stable to probing during arthroscopy.

Fig. 2. Stable OCD lesion. Shadow in low light demarcates the border of the lesion.

Several authors have also described classification systems for OCD of the knee for MRI.[6,12–18] These classifications do share some similarities. Many of the existing classification systems describe intact articular cartilage for stable or low-graded lesions.[6,12–19] Similarly, multiple authors also agree that high-signal intensity between the parent bone and progeny fragment indicates lesion instability,[6,12–17] although in some cases this higher signal may indicate healing or fibrous tissue at the interface.[12] However, arthroscopic visualization remains the reference standard for determining the stability of an OCD lesion of the knee.

Arthroscopic Classification Systems for OCD of the Knee

In 1979, Guhl[20] published a report on the arthroscopic treatment of OCD. This report began with a statement that arthroscopy should first begin with classification of the lesion. Guhl described 4 variations of lesions: intact lesions, early separation, partial detachment, and craters and loose bodies (**Table 1**). Although Guhl's classification was simple, it provided a foundation on which others have built more comprehensive systems classifying OCD of the knee. This classification also identified an important aspect of OCD lesions: delineating between stable (intact lesions) or unstable (separation and eventual loose body formation). This distinction between stable and unstable is present in many of the subsequent classification systems.

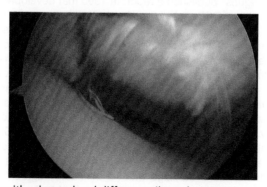

Fig. 3. OCD lesion with advanced and diffuse cartilage changes.

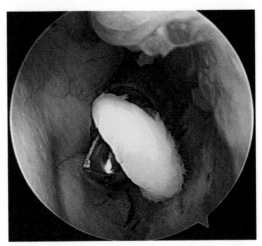

Fig. 4. Loose OCD body in the knee joint.

Ewing and Voto[21] published a similar report in 1988, also describing a system for classifying OCD lesions during arthroscopy. This classification system is remarkably similar to that described by Guhl[20] in 1979, with only minor changes in the description of each stage. According to Ewing and Voto, grade I is classified as an intact lesions, grade II is described as early cartilage separation, grade III is a partially attached lesion, and grade IV is a crater with a loose body (see **Table 1**).

In 1990, Johnson and colleagues[22] described different diagnostic groupings of OCD lesions, and included references to Smillie[23] during his discussion of these groups. Each distinct group was based on integrity of the cartilage and mobility of the fragment. Classifications were given at the time of diagnostic arthroscopy, and the designated classification influenced the surgical treatment. A lesion could be classified into 3 main groupings: articular cartilage intact, articular cartilage separated (unstable), and fragment completely loose (see **Table 1**). For those classified as having intact articular cartilage, the lesion could further be identified as either a stable fragment or a fragment that was mobile with compression. Unstable lesions, or those with separated articular cartilage, could further be classified into being a fragment in situ, or a hinged or partially attached fragment. Lesions designated as completely loose fragments were not further classified.

Nelson and colleagues[6] published a report in 1990 that developed an arthroscopic grading system for knee OCD lesions, similar to those discussed previously.[24] The system consisted of grades 0 through 4. grade 0 was described as a normal lesion. Grade 1 lesions had a focal area of cartilage softening, fibrillation, and fissuring without a definable fragment. Grade 2 lesions presented with a breach in the cartilage with a nondisplaceable fragment. Grade 3 lesions were characterized by a displaceable fragment attached by a flap of articular cartilage. Finally, grade 4 lesions were described as a completely detached fragment or loose body within the joint (see **Table 1**).

In 1991, Dipaola and colleagues[14] expanded on the radiographic classification of Berndt and Harty.[7] They described a method for classifying OCD lesions during arthroscopy and attempted to correlate these findings on MRI. This classification system included 4 stages of lesions. Stage I lesions were defined as having irregularity and softening of the articular cartilage with no definable fragment. Stage II lesions had a breach of the articular cartilage and a definable fragment that was not

Table 1
Arthroscopic classification systems for OCD of the knee

Author, Year	Journal	Stage	Description of Stage
Brittberg et al,[26] 2003	J Bone Joint Surg Am	ICRS OCD I	Stable lesions with a continuous but softened area covered by intact cartilage
		ICRS OCD II	Lesions with partial discontinuity that are stable when probed
		ICRS OCD III	Lesions with a complete discontinuity that are not yet dislocated (dead in situ)
		ICRS OCD IV	Empty defects and those with a dislocated fragment or a loose fragment within the bed
		Subgroup I–IVB	Defects that are >10 mm in depth
Chen, 2013[13]	Eur J Radiol	Stage I	Intact but partially soft and cartilage
		Stage II	Overlying cartilage fissure
		Stage III	Exposed bone or attached fragment
		Stage IV	Partially detached fragment
		Stage V	Carters with loose bodies
Dipaola et al,[14] 1991	Arthroscopy	Stage I	Irregularity and softening of the articular cartilage; no definable fragment
		Stage II	Articular cartilage breached, definable fragment, not displaceable
		Stage III	Articular cartilage breached, definable fragment, displaceable, but attached by some overlying articular cartilage
		Stave IV	Loose body
Ewing & Voto,[21] 1988	Arthroscopy	Grade I	Intact lesion
		Grade II	Early cartilage separation
		Grade III	Partially attached lesion
		Grade IV	Crater lesion with loose body
Guhl,[20] 1979	Orthop Clin North Am	Type I	Intact lesion
		Type II	Early separation
		Type III	Partial detachment
		Type IV	Craters and loose bodies
Johnson et al,[22] 1990	Arthroscopy	Articular cartilage intact	Fragment stable
			Fragment mobile with compression
		Articular cartilage separated (unstable)	Fragment in situ
			Fragment hinged (partially intact)
		Fragment completely loose	
Nelson et al,[6] 1990	J Comput Assist Tom	Grade 0	Normal
		Grade 1	A focal area of cartilaginous softening, fibrillation, and fissuring without a definable fragment
		Grade 2	A breach in the cartilage with a nondisplaceable fragment
		Grade 3	Displaceable fragment attached by a flap of articular cartilage
		Grade 4	A completely detached fragment or loose body within the joint

(continued on next page)

Table 1 (continued)			
Author, Year	**Journal**	**Stage**	**Description of Stage**
O'Connor et al,[25] 2002	*J Bone Joint Surg Br*	Grade I	Irregularity and softening of cartilage; no fissure; no definable fragment
		Grade II	Articular cartilage breached; not displaceable
		Grade III	Definable fragment displaceable, but still attached partially by some cartilage (ie, a flap lesion)
		Grade IV	Loose body and defect of the articular surface

displaceable. Stage III lesions also had a breach of the articular cartilage with a definable fragment that was displaceable but was attached by some overlying articular cartilage. Stage IV lesions were loose bodies (see **Table 1**).

O'Connor and colleagues[25] used a classification system attributed to Guhl[20] in a study published in 2002. However, a review of the classification system O'Connor and colleagues[25] described found that the descriptive language in this system differed from the original classification published by Guhl.[20] The classification system used by O'Connor and colleagues attempted to correlate MRI findings with arthroscopic findings; their arthroscopy classification consisted of 4 stages. Stage I lesions were defined as having irregularity and softening of the (articular) cartilage, with no fissure or definable fragment. Stage II lesions had a breach of the articular cartilage and (a definable fragment) was not displaceable. Stage III lesions also had a breach of the articular cartilage with a definable fragment that was displaceable but still partially attached by some cartilage (ie, flap lesion). Stage IV lesions were loose bodies with a defect of the articular surface (see **Table 1**).

Recognizing a need for more standardized and universally accepted systems for classifying articular cartilage defects, the International Cartilage Repair Society (ICRS) published a series of classifications systems, one of which was specific to OCD of the knee (**Fig. 5**). This system, reported by Brittberg and Winalski[26] in 2003, consisted of 4 stages of OCD lesions, with a subgroup of I through IVB for lesions that were greater that 10 mm in depth. ICRS OCD I designation was given to stable lesions with a continuous but softened area covered by intact cartilage. Lesions with partial discontinuity that are stable when probed were classified as ICRS OCD II. ICRS OCD III designation was given to lesions with complete discontinuity that are not yet dislocated (*dead in situ*). ICRS OCD IV was described as empty defects and those with a dislocated fragment or a loose fragment within the bed (see **Table 1**).

In 2013, Chen and colleagues[13] described a classification system developed from modifying a system described by the American Sports Medicine Institute. This classification system consisted of 5 stages. Stage I lesions had intact but partially soft cartilage. Classification of stage II was given to lesions with an overlying cartilage fissure. Stage III lesions had exposed bone or an attached fragment. Partially detached fragments were classified as Stage IV. Stage V lesions were craters with loose bodies (see **Table 1**).

DISCUSSION

Several inconsistencies were identified among the articles reviewed. Guhl[20] described one of the first classification systems for OCD of the knee during arthroscopy, and

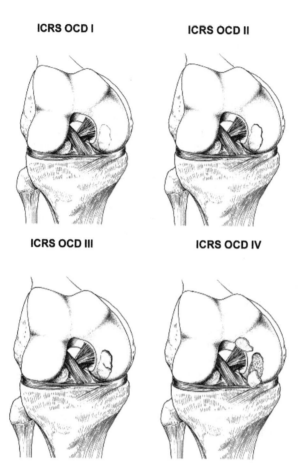

ICRS OCD I   **ICRS OCD II**

ICRS OCD III   **ICRS OCD IV**

Fig. 5. ICRS classification of OCD-Lesions (osteochondritis dissecans). (Images kindly provided by the International Cartilage Repair Society. ICRS Clinical Cartilage Injury Evaluation System. Available at: http://www.cartilage.org/?pid5223; Accessed November 2, 2013; with permission.)

therefore it is accepted that many of the subsequently described classification systems would have some similarities. However, the classification system described by Ewing and Voto[21] is very similar in the number of stages of the OCD lesion and the description of each stage. Because it was an independently described classification, it was included in the present review.

The study published by O'Connor and colleagues[25] indicated that the classification system by Guhl[20] was used. However, a comparison of their classification system and the original system described by Guhl found that they were not identical. Furthermore, the classification described by O'Connor and colleagues was remarkably similar to that described by Dipaola and colleagues[14] 11 years prior. This discrepancy illustrates the lack of rigor used in methodological reporting of some of these studies. Although a detailed methodology is not necessary to report a classification system, it may be requisite if such a system is to become the standard tool for assessing OCD lesions of the knee during arthroscopic surgery.

Chen and colleagues[13] reported that the classification system described in their paper was modified from the staging system of the American Sports Medicine

Institute. However, the authors failed to provide citation for the staging system they modified. A review of the literature found an article published by Baumgarten and colleagues[27] out of the American Sports Medicine Institute that described a classification system for OCD lesions of the elbow capitellum that the present authors identified as being similar to that described by Chen and colleagues.[13]

Arthroscopic classification systems contain many consistencies, providing potential for the development of a universal system. In the literature reviewed, most classifications identify the earliest stage of OCD as a softening of the site when probed, whereas the articular cartilage remains intact.[6,13,14,22,25,26] The intermediate stages are commonly regarded as fissuring or a partial disruption in the cartilage that remains stable. The final classification stages involve a partially detached fragment progressing to become a loose body within the joint. Although agreement between studies does exist, further research and collaboration is still needed to reach a consensus on the necessary specificity of the steps to accurately describe OCD lesions during arthroscopy.

SUMMARY

Multiple systems have been described over the past several decades for classifying OCD of the knee during arthroscopic surgery. However, no single classification system has been universally accepted and routinely used. Although this lack of uniformity could be caused by several factors, one central issue identified in this review was that no study assessed the inter-rater and intra-rater reliability of their classification system. Reliability testing will need to be completed to determine the overall utility of a classification system. Future research should be performed in this area to establish a standard classification system for OCD of the knee during arthroscopy that shows high inter-rater and intra-rater reliability. A future system should include a description of the lesion's articular cartilage contour and stability/integrity, and a gross overall description of the lesion.

REFERENCES

1. Edmonds EW, Shea KG. Osteochondritis dissecans: editorial comment. Clin Orthop Relat Res 2013;471(4):1105–6.
2. Cahill BR. Osteochondritis dissecans of the knee: treatment of juvenile and adult forms. J Am Acad Orthop Surg 1995;3:237–47.
3. Kessler JI, Nikizad H, Shea KG, et al. The demographics and epidemiology of osteochondritis dissecans of the knee in children and adolescents. Am J Sports Med 2013; [Epub ahead of print].
4. Linden B. The incidence of osteochondritis dissecans in the condyles of the femur. Acta Orthop Scand 1976;47:664–7.
5. Mesgarzadeh M, Sapega AA, Bonakdarpour A, et al. Osteochondritis dissecans: analysis of mechanical stability with radiography, scintigraphy, and MR imaging. Radiology 1987;165:775–80.
6. Nelson DW, DiPaola J, Colville M, et al. Osteochondritis dissecans of the talus and knee: prospective comparison of MR and arthroscopic classifications. J Comput Assist Tomogr 1990;14:804–8.
7. Berndt AL, Harty M. Transchondral fractures (osteochondritis dissecans) of the talus. J Bone Joint Surg Am 1959;41:988–1020.
8. Kocher MS, Micheli LJ, Yaniv M, et al. Functional and radiographic outcome of juvenile osteochondritis dissecans of the knee treated with transarticular arthroscopic drilling. Am J Sports Med 2001;29:562–6.

9. Rodegerdts U, Gleissner B. Langzeiterfabrung mit der operativen therapie der osteochondrosis dissecans des kniegelenkes. Orthop Prax 1981;8:612–22.

10. Lefort G, Moyen B, Beaufils P, et al. Osteochondritis dissecans of the femoral condyles: report of 892 cases. Rev Chir Orthop Reparatrice Appar Mot 2006; 92:2S97–141.

11. Satake H, Takahara M, Harada M, et al. Preoperative imaging criteria for unstable osteochondritis dissecans of the capitellum. Clin Orthop Relat Res 2013;471(4): 1137–43.

12. Bohndorf K. Osteochondritis (osteochondrosis) dissecans: a review and new MRI classification. Eur Radiol 1998;8:103–12.

13. Chen CH, Liu YS, Chou PH, et al. MR grading system of osteochondritis dissecans lesions: comparison with arthroscopy. Eur J Radiol 2013;82:518–25.

14. Dipaola JD, Nelson DW, Colville MR. Characterizing osteochondral lesions by magnetic resonance imaging. Arthroscopy 1991;7:101–4.

15. Hefti F, Beguiristain J, Krauspe R, et al. Osteochondritis dissecans: a multicenter study of the European Pediatric Orthopedic Society. J Pediatr Orthop B 1999;8: 231–45.

16. Hughes JA, Cook JV, Churchill MA, et al. Juvenile osteochondritis dissecans: a 5-year review of the natural history using clinical and MRI evaluation. Pediatr Radiol 2003;33:410–7.

17. Schulz JF, Chambers HG. Juvenile osteochondritis dissecans of the knee: current concepts in diagnosis and management. Instr Course Lect 2013;62:455–67.

18. Taranow WS, Bisignani GA, Towers JD, et al. Retrograde drilling of osteochondral lesions of the medial talar dome. Foot Ankle Int 1999;20:474–80.

19. Kramer J, Stiglbauer R, Engel A, et al. MR contrast arthrography (MRA) in osteochondrosis dissecans. J Comput Assist Tomogr 1992;16:254–60.

20. Guhl JF. Arthroscopic treatment of osteochondritis dissecans: preliminary report. Orthop Clin North Am 1979;10:671–83.

21. Ewing JW, Voto SJ. Arthroscopic surgical management of osteochondritis dissecans of the knee. Arthroscopy 1988;4:37–40.

22. Johnson LL, Uitvlugt G, Austin MD, et al. Osteochondritis dissecans of the knee: arthroscopic compression screw fixation. Arthroscopy 1990;6:179–89.

23. Smillie IS. Injuries of the knee joint. 4th edition. Edinburgh (United Kingdom): E. & S. Livingstone Ltd; 1975.

24. Pritsch M, Horoshovski H, Farine I. Arthroscopic treatment of osteochondral lesions of the talus. J Bone Joint Surg Am 1986;68:862–5.

25. O'Connor MA, Palaniappan M, Khan N, et al. Osteochondritis dissecans of the knee in children. A comparison of MRI and arthroscopic findings. J Bone Joint Surg Br 2002;84:258–62.

26. Brittberg M, Winalski CS. Evaluation of cartilage injuries and repair. J Bone Joint Surg Am 2003;85(Suppl 2):58–69.

27. Baumgarten TE, Andrews JR, Satterwhite YE. The arthroscopic classification and treatment of osteochondritis dissecans of the capitellum. Am J Sports Med 1998; 26:520–3.

Emerging Genetic Basis of Osteochondritis Dissecans

J. Tyler Bates[a], John C. Jacobs Jr, BS[b], Kevin G. Shea, MD[c,d],
Julia Thom Oxford, PhD[a],*

KEYWORDS

- Osteochondritis dissecans • Osteochondrosis • Genome-wide association study
- Osteoarthritis • Single nucleotide polymorphism • Human • Equine • Swine

KEY POINTS

- PTH1R is a strong candidate gene for OCD, identified in both horses and pigs, indicating the potential for involvement of pathways that mediate transition from cartilage to bone during endochondral ossification and growth plate maturation.
- Genes identified include secreted proteins of the extracellular matrix and the genes encoding proteins that mediate the cellular secretory pathway.
- The identified genetic loci may also indicate a higher risk for osteoarthritis.

INTRODUCTION

Osteochondritis dissecans (OCD) is a focal idiopathic alteration of subchondral bone with risk for instability and disruption of adjacent articular cartilage that may result in premature osteoarthritis (OA).[1] This condition is commonly found in horses, pigs, dogs, and humans.[2] König[3] first used the term OCD to describe a condition that causes the formation of loose bodies in the joints of young individuals without arthritis or trauma. Although more than 100 years have passed since König[3] described OCD, little knowledge exists of the specific etiology and pathogenesis of this disease. Many etiologic theories have been proposed for the onset and progression of OCD, including trauma, diet, rapid growth, anatomic characteristics, lack of blood supply, necrosis of subchondral bone, and heredity (recently reviewed in Refs. [4–8]). Recent experiments have provided additional information regarding the underlying genetic traits that may predispose an individual to OCD.

[a] Department of Biological Sciences, Biomolecular Research Center, Musculoskeletal Research Institute, Boise State University, 1910 University Drive, Boise, ID 83725, USA; [b] University of Utah School of Medicine, 30 North 1900 East, Salt Lake City, UT 84132, USA; [c] St. Luke's Sports Medicine, St. Luke's Health System, St. Luke's Children's Hospital, 600 North Robbins Road, Suite 400, Boise, ID 83702, USA; [d] Department of Orthopedics, University of Utah, 590 Wakara Way, Salt Lake City, UT 84108, USA
* Corresponding author.
E-mail address: joxford@boisestate.edu

Clin Sports Med 33 (2014) 199–220
http://dx.doi.org/10.1016/j.csm.2013.11.004
0278-5919/14/$ – see front matter © 2014 Elsevier Inc. All rights reserved.

König's[3] original description included inflammation as a contributor to the formation of OCD lesions and "joint mice." However, recent research has suggested that inflammation is not involved in the etiology of OCD, and thus should be referred to as osteochondrosis.[4,8,9] In the clinical and research settings, osteochondrosis represents a larger range of disorders than the original condition described by König.[3,8] Although the term OCD is used in human disease, much of the animal literature uses the term osteochondrosis to describe what may actually be the same condition.

In humans, OCD can affect both juveniles and adults,[10] although onset is typically in skeletally immature patients. If untreated, OCD can lead to OA as the age of the individual progresses.[11–13] Although both surgical and nonsurgical treatments are available for patients with OCD,[14] a better understanding of the pathogenesis of OCD and the underlying genetics may provide opportunities for better diagnosis and additional treatment options.[14]

Osteochondrosis has been investigated primarily in horses and pigs. Osteochondrosis is the leading cause of lameness and decreased performance in young athletic horses.[15] Osteochondrosis is also considered the leading cause of leg weakness in pigs.[16,17] The most extensive analysis of genetic association has been completed for the disease in horses and pigs, to date.

Much of the previous research on the pathogenesis of OCD in humans has been through histologic analysis of bone samples. A recent review by Shea and colleagues[4] found an overall lack of histologic OCD research, with varying methodologies and findings among the studies reviewed. One issue inherent in histologic analysis of tissue samples is that only a limited number of different proteins or markers can be tested and samples may at best represent end-stage or advanced stages of the disease. Tissue samples are available only during certain surgical procedures, and thus it can be difficult to obtain large or multiple sample sizes. Furthermore, biopsy specimens are unlikely to represent early stages of OCD.

Previous studies have analyzed candidate genes and their association with the onset of OCD[18–20]; however, these efforts have been limited. With improved techniques and decreasing costs for genetic studies, the opportunity for genome-wide association studies (GWAS) and single-nucleotide polymorphism (SNP) studies has become available. The purpose of this review was twofold: first, to review the most recent literature on GWAS and SNP studies on OCD and osteochondrosis, and second, to identify patterns within the genes of interest to serve as a guide for further investigation into the etiology of OCD.

In a GWAS study, subjects are evaluated based on physical traits and then genotyped. The traits are compared with the gene sequences by a computer program, which calculates the correlation. Markers are designed and used to split the DNA at intervals that span the chromosomes. The markers are designed to identify SNPs where the genetic code tends to vary by a single base pair across individuals. Based on the locations of SNPs with high statistical significance (call rate), nearby genes can be identified as possible genes of interest for the selected trait. The gene regions with possible linkage to the trait are referenced as quantitative trait loci (QTL).

METHODS

A Medline search was performed in March of 2013 to identify relevant genetic studies of OCD in all animals and humans (**Fig. 1**). Searches were performed for both "osteochondritis dissecans" and "osteochondrosis" because of the historical interchange of terms with the following key words: "osteochondritis dissecans AND single nucleotide polymorphism," "osteochondrosis AND single nucleotide polymorphism,"

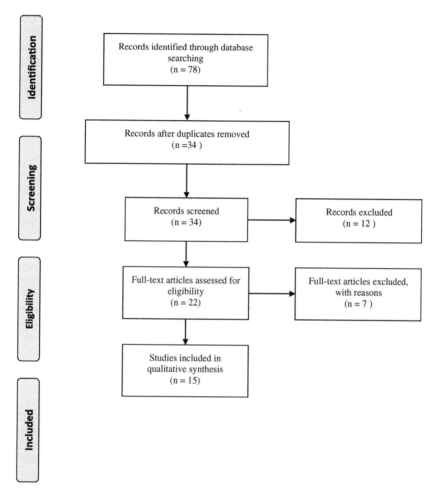

Fig. 1. PRISMA flow diagram. *Preferred Reporting Items for Systematic Reviews and Meta-Analyses* guidelines were used to select journal articles for inclusion and review. (*Adapted from* Moher D, Liberati A, Tetzlaff J, et al. The PRISMA Group. Preferred Reporting Items for Systematic Reviews and Meta-Analyses: The PRISMA Statement. PLoS Med 2009;6:e1000097.)

"osteochondritis dissecans AND genome-wide association study," "osteochondrosis AND genome-wide association study," "osteochondritis dissecans AND genome," "osteochondrosis AND genome," "osteochondritis dissecans AND cell signaling," "osteochondrosis AND cell signaling," "osteochondritis dissecans AND quantitative trait loci," and "osteochondrosis AND quantitative trait loci." All searches were completed with an English language filter.

Duplicate articles were removed and abstracts were screened according to the following inclusion criteria: experimental research performing GWAS, studies of SNP, or refinements to previously completed articles. Articles that did not meet inclusion criteria were heritability reports, cell culture or tissue studies of genes, or mRNA expression. Studies investigating SNPs within selected genes were also discarded because of the high degree of specificity of the SNP location.

Twenty-two articles were identified after screening. Of those, 7 were excluded, which resulted in the inclusion of 15 in the current review. Of those 15 articles, one studied human OCD with a genome-wide linkage analysis, 12 studies were in equines, and 2 were genetic studies in swine. All articles were published between 2000 and 2013. A description of OCD or osteochondrosis, experimental methods, and results are found in the following sections, organized by the species. The results from GWAS are summarized in **Tables 1** and **2**.

REVIEW
Human

OCD in humans is primarily found in the knee, elbow, or ankle of adolescents. The subchondral bone is affected, leading to disruption of articular cartilage and possible formation of osteochondral fragments. Familial cases of OCD were recently characterized by osteochondritic lesions in different joints, short stature, and early OA due to mutations in the aggrecan gene.[19]

Stattin and colleagues[19] studied 53 members of 5 generations of a Swedish family with inherited OCD, 15 of whom were diagnosed with OCD by magnetic resonance imaging (MRI) or X-ray. Blood samples were taken from the 53 subjects and genomic DNA was extracted from white blood cells. Genotyping was completed on 38 of the individuals using 400 microsatellite markers, which spanned all autosomes with an average spacing of 10 cM. Linkage was then analyzed using MCLINK from Myriad Genetics (Salt Lake City, UT). A significant polymorphic marker was found on chromosome 15, revealing aggrecan (*ACAN*) to be a gene of interest. Further work was completed to test the mutated *ACAN* gene in vivo.

Equine

Osteochondrosis normally affects young horses at 5 to 8 months of age.[21] Osteochondrosis in horses is defined as a disturbance of endochondral ossification at the epiphyseal growth plate. Disturbance during differentiation, development, and vascular invasion of the growth plate leads to alterations of the joint, formation of cartilage flaps, or osseous fragments.[22] Osteochondrosis is primarily diagnosed via radiography, and is usually not identified until the formation of the loose bony or osteochondral fragments. Much of the recent literature identifies a disease stage in which bony fragments are present, referred to as osteochondrosis dissecans.[8] Teyssedre and colleagues[23] referred to osteochondrosis as a generic term for OCD and bone cysts. Although osteochondrosis is present in many different joints in the horse, most research has focused on the tarsocrural (hock) joint because of the high incidence and defined diagnosis methods.[24] Evidence for heritability has been found at frequencies between 0.2 and 0.64, depending on the location of the osteochondrosis lesion and the breed of the horse.[22] Osteochondrosis is economically important and affects animal welfare in a significant manner.[25]

After review, 12 articles were deemed relevant.[2,21,23–32] Four of the included articles[28–31] were refinements to the work done in Dierks and colleagues.[27] Two refinement studies were also completed by Wittwer and associates[25,32] on the work of Wittwer and colleagues.[21] In total, 6 studies completed GWAS to identify candidate genes responsible for osteochondrosis, and 6 studies were conducted on specific gene regions for fine mapping of previous work. In all studies, horses were diagnosed with osteochondrosis via radiography and scored for severity.

Corbin and colleagues[26] had 162 case horses with osteochondrosis and 168 control subjects. Dierks and colleagues' studies[27–32] used 76 horses with osteochondrosis and 28 unaffected horses for controls. Orr and colleagues[24] used 90 osteochondrotic

Table 1
Results from equine GWAS

Author(s), Year	Journal	Population Size	Number of SNP Markers	Map Length	Equine SNP Location	Corresponding Genes	Additional Genes from Refinement Studies
Corbin et al,[26] 2012	Mamm Genome	330	40,180	All autosomes	Chr 3 at 88.49 cM	—	
Dierks et al,[27] 2007	Mamm Genome	104	260	All autosomes	Chr 2 at 22.00–43.41 cM	Matrilin 1 (MATN1)	Neurochondrin (NCDN), Ficolin3 (FCN3), and Mitochondrial trans-2-enoyl CoA reductase (MECR)
					Chr 4 at 7.70–24.30 cM	Laminin (LAMB1)	Hyaluronoglucosaminidase (HYAL) family
					Chr 5 at 79.30 cM	Solute carrier family 35 member D1 (SLC35D1)	Collage type XXIV $\alpha 1$ (COL24A1)
					Chr 16 at 33.00–45.00 cM	Parathyroid hormone receptor (PTH1R)	
					Chr 18 at 74.94–82.25 cM	—	Parathyroid hormone 2 receptor (PTH2R)
Lykkjen et al,[2] 2010	Anim Genet	162	41,170	All autosomes	Chr 1 at 139 cM	—	
					Chr 3 at 113 cM	—	
					Chr 5 at 42, 77, and 79 cM	Chloride channel, calcium activated, family member 4 (CLCA4); Collagen type XXIV $\alpha 1$ (COL24A1)	
					Chr 10 at 80 cM	LOC10007351	
					Chr 18 at 59 cM	TBC1 domain family member 22A (TBC1D22A)	
					Chr 28 at 43 cM		

(continued on next page)

Table 1
(continued)

Author(s), Year	Journal	Population Size	Number of SNP Markers	Map Length	Equine SNP Location	Corresponding Genes	Additional Genes from Refinement Studies
Orr et al,[24] 2012	Anim Genet	201	45,586	All autosomes	Chr 3 at 105 cM Chr 10 at 48 cM Chr 16 at 47 cM Chr 21 at 11 cM Chr 31 at 22 cM	— — — — —	
Teyssedre et al,[23] 2012	J AnimSci	525	41,249	All autosomes	Chr 3 at 105 cM Chr 13 at 9 cM Chr 14 at 73 cM Chr 15 at 87 cM	— — — —	
Wittwer et al,[21,22] 2007	Anim Genet	117	157	All autosomes and X-chr	Chr 1 at 150.0–194.2 cM Chr 4 at 7.8–38.0 cM	Lectin, galactoside—binding soluble, 3 (LGALS3) Calcitonin gene—related peptide—receptor component protein (RCP9); Calneuron 1 (CALN1)	
					Chr 4 at 70.0 cM	Interleukin 6 (IL6)	Acyloxyacyl hydrolase (AOAH)
					Chr 18 at 45.9–87.6 cM	Collagen type III α1 (COL3A1); Collagen type V α2 (COL5A2); Frizzled-related protein (FRZB)	Xin actin-binding repeat containing 2 (XIRP2)
					Chr 25 at 30.1 cM	Collagen type V α1 (COL5A1); Collagen XXVII α1 (COL27A1)	

Identified genes and research methods in horses are outlined by article.
Abbreviations: Chr, chromosome; SNP, single-nucleotide polymorphism; —, no corresponding gene identified for the designated locus.

Table 2
Results of GWAS from swine

Author(s), Year	Journal	Population Size	Number of SNP Markers	Map Length	Pig SNP Location	Corresponding Human Genes
Andersson-Eklund et al,[34] 2000	Genet Res	195	236	2300 cM	Chr 5 at 51 cm	Cartilage homeoprotein 1 (CART1)
					Chr 13 at 64 cm	PIT1, Parathyroid hormone receptor (PTHR)
Laenoi et al,[17] 2011	Genet Sel Evol	310	79 microsatellites, 3 biallelic markers	2588.7 cM	Chr 2 at 14 cM	—
					Chr 3 at 13 cM	—
					Chr 6 at 61 cM	—
					Chr 10 at 70 cM	—
					Chr 14 at 0 cM	—

Identified genes and research methods in pigs are outlined by article.
Abbreviations: Chr, chromosome; SNP, single-nucleotide polymorphism; —, no corresponding gene identified for the designated locus.

horses with 111 controls. In the research performed by Lykkjen and colleagues,[2] 80 horses with osteochondrosis were compared with 82 control horses. The largest sample size was used by Teyssedre and colleagues,[23] with 262 affected horses and 263 healthy horses for control. The initial work done by Wittwer and colleagues[21] had 96 osteochondrotic horses and 18 controls. Thirty-two affected and 64 healthy horses were included in studies by Wittwer and colleagues,[32] whereas 96 horses were used in Wittwer and colleagues.[25] Corbin and colleagues[26] tested Thoroughbred horses in their study. Hanoverian Warmblood horses were used in 5 of the studies.[27–31] South German Coldblood horses were used in 3 studies.[21,25,32] Dutch Warmblood horses, French trotter horses, and Norwegian Standardbred trotters were studied.[2,23,24]

Genotyping was accomplished in 4 of the articles by using the Illumina Equine SNP50 BeadChip with 54,602 SNPs.[2,23,24,26] Each of the articles applied quality control measures, decreasing the amount of tested SNPs to 40,180,[26] 45,586 with an average call rate of 99.8%,[24] 41,170 with a minimum call rate of 95%,[2] and 41,249 with a minimum call rate of 98%.[23] Initial genotyping was completed with 172 highly polymorphic microsatellites by Dierks and colleagues,[27] with 88 additional microsatellites added for putative QTLs established in the first scan for a total of 260 microsatellite markers. Refinement studies added 49, 34, 11, and 37 new microsatellites on chromosomes 5, 16, 18, and 2, respectively.[29–31]

Statistical analysis was completed using MERLIN (multipoint engine for rapid likelihood inference) software (freeware can be downloaded from sph.umich.edu/csg/abecasis/software.html) by Dierks and colleagues[27–30] and Wittwer and colleagues.[21,25,32] Lykkjen and colleagues[2] used the whole-genome association analysis toolset PLINK (freely available at http://pngu.mgh.harvard.edu/~purcell/plink/) for statistical calculations. Orr and colleagues[24] used GENABEL (free software at genabel.org) and HAPLOSTATS (freely available at inside-r.org/packages/haplostats) for their analysis work. REMFL90 software (freeware from nce.ads.uga.edu) was used by Teyssedre and colleagues[23] for statistical analysis calculations. A summary of results is shown in **Table 1**.

Corbin and colleagues[26] identified UDP-glucose dehydrogenase (*UGDH*) as a possible related gene to osteochondrosis. Dierks and colleagues[27] identified connections between SNPs found in their research and human genes. The genes identified were matrilin 1 (*MATN1*), laminin (*LAMB1*), solute carrier family 35 (*SLC35D1*), and parathyroid hormone receptor (*PTH1R*). Collagen type XXIV alpha 1 (*COL24A1*) was identified as a functional candidate gene in Lampe and colleagues.[29] The hyaluronoglucosaminidase gene family members were identified as candidates in Lampe and colleagues.[30] Refinement done by Lampe and colleagues[31] found parathyroid hormone 2 receptor (*PTH2R*) to be associated with osteochondrosis. The gene neurochondrin (*NCDN*) was concluded to be the functional candidate gene on ECA2 by Dierks and colleagues.[28] Lykkjen and colleagues[2] found LOC100073151, chloride channel calcium-activated family member 4 (*CLCA4*), *COL24A1*, F-box protein 25 (*FBXO25*), and TBC1 domain family member 22A (*TBC1D22A*) to be possible genes contributing to osteochondrosis in the horse. Lectin galactoside-binding soluble 3 (*LGALS3*), frizzled-related protein (*FRZB*), collagen type III alpha 1 (*COL3A1*), collagen type V alpha 2 (*COL5A2*), collagen type V alpha 1 (*COL5A2*), collagen type XXVII alpha 1 (*COL27A1*), calcitonin gene-related peptide-receptor component protein (*RCP9*), calneuron 1 (*CALN1*), and interleukin 6 (*IL6*) were also identified as candidate genes.[21] Wittwer and colleagues[32] identified *AOAH* and *PTH1R* as other possible genes. Xin actin-binding repeat containing 2 (*XIRP2*) was shown to be a strong candidate gene.

Swine

Osteochondrosis in swine is considered to be a generalized skeletal disease characterized by disturbed bone formation, cartilage retention, or necrosis of cartilage canal in articular cartilage.[33,34] Osteochondrosis is the primary cause of leg weakness in swine, impacting the fitness and longevity of animals.[17] Previous studies have analyzed the relationship among growth rate, weight, and diet with osteochondrosis.[8] Leg weakness is a general term that integrates many different diseases and conditions and may not be limited specifically to osteochondrosis. Heritability of osteochondrosis varies by breed but has been found to range from 0.06 to 0.5.[17]

Laenoi and colleagues[17] established a genetic link to leg weakness and osteochondrosis. They identified SNPs related to bone mineral density in addition to leg weakness and osteochondrosis, and performed genotyping with 79 microsatellites and 3 biallelic markers (a higher tolerance marker type) for an average marker interval of 31.57 cM. Additional SNPs in the COL10A1 and MMP3 loci were included, due to the relevance to cartilage quality. Andersson-Ekland and colleagues[34] focused on phenotypic attributes and osteochondrosis. They used 236 markers across all autosomes. Leg weakness and osteochondrosis were also assessed from histologic evaluation. A summary of findings is presented in **Table 2**.

QTLs related to osteochondrosis were found on chromosomes 5 and 13 at 51 cM and 64 cM, respectively, by Andersson-Eklund and colleagues.[34] The SNP at chromosome 5 was located between interferon-γ and insulin-like growth factor-1 with homology to human chromosome 12q14-q24 and the gene for cartilage homeoprotein 1 (CART1). Homology also exists in the region of the QTL on chromosome 13 for pituitary-specific positive transcription factor 1 (PIT1) and parathyroid hormone receptor (PTH1R) genes. Laenoi and colleagues[17] found QTLs on chromosomes 2, 3, 6, 10, and 14. The QTLs were located at 14 cM on chromosome 2, 13 cM on chromosome 3, 61 cM on chromosome 6, 70 cM on chromosome 10, and 0 cM for chromosome 14. Genes located at these identified polymorphisms are yet to be determined.

DISCUSSION

OCD in humans affects the subchondral bone, primarily in the knee, elbow, or ankle leading to disruption of articular cartilage and possible formation of osteochondral fragments.[14] Etiology in humans may be related to several other factors, including trauma, ischemia, and disrupted endochondral ossification.[4,12,35–37] In equine osteochondrosis, endochondral ossification of the epiphyseal growth plate is disrupted, leading to the formation of the loose bony osteochondral fragments. Different joints are affected with the highest incidence in the tarsocrural joint. Evidence supports inherited genetic traits underlying osteochondrosis in equines. Osteochondrosis in swine is characterized by disturbed bone formation, cartilage retention, or necrosis of cartilage canals in calcified cartilage.[33,34] Heritability of osteochondrosis in swine varies by breed; however, the argument for the existence of genetic factors is strong.

Candidate Genes Cluster into Distinct Groups

Candidate genes were identified in GWAS and through additional refinement of these studies. Analysis of these genes indicates a high prevalence for those encoding secreted extracellular matrix proteins, and those playing a role in the secretory pathway. Additionally, a cluster of genes regulating the differentiation and maturation of the growth plate was also observed. Notably, extracellular matrix molecules and parathyroid hormone signaling were identified in multiple studies and by multiple candidate genes.

Extracellular Matrix Proteins

COL24A1 was identified as a candidate gene in the refinement study completed by Lampe and colleagues[29] and by the GWAS analyzed by Lykkjen and colleagues.[2] Wittwer and colleagues[21] found COL3A1, COL5A1, COL5A2, COL10A1, and COL27A1 to be significantly associated with incidence of osteochondrosis in horses. Additional extracellular matrix molecules included MATN1, LAMB1, and ACAN. Genes involved in extracellular matrix turnover include hyaluronoglucosaminidase (HYAL) and matrix metalloproteinase 3 (MMP3).

The hyaluronidases comprise a family of lysosomal β-endoglucosidases that are responsible for the turnover of hyaluronan, a ubiquitous extracellular maxtrix glycosaminoglycan, by cleaving internal β-1,4 linkages. Six hyaluronidase genes have been identified in humans,[38,39] clustered at chromosomal locations 3p21.3 (HYAL-1, HYAL-2, and HYAL-3) and at chr 7q31.3 (HYAL-4, HYALP1, and SPAM-1). Cartilage has been shown to express mRNA encoding HYAL-1, HYAL-2, and HYAL-3.[40] TCF/Lef binding sites have been identified within the promoter regions, indicating a link to the Wnt signaling pathway.[41] Tissue remodeling and growth during skeletal development relies on HYAL family member function.

Matrilins (MATNs) are a family of 4 oligomeric extracellular matrix proteins. Each family member contains a von Willebrand factor A domain, epidermal growth factor–like domains, and coiled–coil domains.[42] Mutations in MATNs have been associated with osteochondrodysplasias, including multiple epiphyseal dysplasia[43–47] and OA.[48–51]

More than 13,000 articles are indexed in Medline relating to cartilage and collagen, 44 of which address the connection between collagen and osteochondrosis. An additional 2500+ studies report a connection between collagen and OA. COL24A1 is described as a fibril diameter regulator with specific functions at specific sites for fibrillogenesis, especially for COL1A1.[52] Skagen and colleagues[53] studied biopsies of osteochondrotic lesions and determined that abnormal collagen fibrils are associated with OCD, with evidence supporting endoplasmic reticulum (ER) stress and an unfolded protein response (UPR) as identified by the extended ER by transmission electron microscopy. Additionally, collagen fibrils in the extracellular matrix appeared abnormal, and evidence of internal cellular accumulation of collagens was evident.[53] A mutation in the gene COL24A1 represents a strong candidate for the effect seen on collagen fibril diameter in the cartilage extracellular matrix, as COL24A1 is known to regulate fibril diameter during fibrillogenesis, is expressed by osteoblasts,[54] and can drive bone development through the transforming growth factor beta (TGF-β) signaling pathway.[55]

Secreted Proteins Associated with Skeletal Dysplasia and/or OCD

Familial cases of OCD have been reported, and in some forms of skeletal dysplasia, conditions resembling OCD had been identified in the patients. This suggests an underlying genetic factor in at least some cases of OCD. Mutations in genes encoding some secreted proteins have been shown to contribute to ER stress. ER stress that induces an unfolded protein response in the cells of the growth plate may contribute to OCD. Cartilage extracellular matrix protein Cartilage Oligomeric Matrix Protein (COMP) causes pseudoachondroplasia (PSACH),[56] and matrilin 3 (MATN3) causes multiple epiphyseal dysplasia (MED),[57] and an unfolded protein response is observed in both cases. Short stature and early-onset OA was associated with familial OCD caused by mutations in *ACAN*.[19]

Other Secreted Proteins

Additional genes encoding secreted proteins identified from GWAS include acyloxyacyl hydrolase (*AOAH*), ficolin 3 (*FCN3*), and chloride channel, calcium activated, family member 4 (*CLCA4*). FCN3, located on human chromosome 1.p36.11, encodes a secreted protein comprising a collagen-like domain and a fibrinogen-like domain. FCN3 has affinity for carbohydrate moieties, is able to activate the complement pathway, and is therefore associated with innate immunity. Although no function for FCN3 in the growth plate has been reported, identification of FCN3 within the serum proteome associated with degenerative scoliosis may indicate a skeletal role.[58] *CLCA4*, located on human chromosome 1p22.3, encodes a calcium-sensitive chloride conductance protein. Initially synthesized as a 125-kDa protein that is restricted to the ER, the protein undergoes specific proteolytic processing to yield 90-kDa and 40-kDa fragments that are secreted and also found associated with the plasma membrane.[59] Acyloxyacyl hydrolase (*AOAH*), located on chromosome 7p14.2, encodes a secreted enzyme capable of hydrolyzing acyloxyacyl-linked fatty acyl chains. A role for AOAH in OCD is currently not known.

Secretory Pathway Proteins

Not only must the extracellular matrix molecules be synthesized by the cell, but they also must be assembled, modified, and secreted properly in order for the extracellular matrix to function properly. Genes that play a role in this process include Solute carrier family 35 member D1 (*SLC35D1*) and UDP-glucose dehydrogenase (*UGDH*). *SLC35D1*, located at human chromosome 1p31.3, is responsible for the glycosylation of proteins within the ER and Golgi compartments of the protein secretion pathway. SLC35D1 transports UDP-glucuronic acid and UDP-N-acetylgalactosamine from the cytoplasm to the lumen of the ER. Chondroitin sulfate (CS) is a critical component of cartilage extracellular matrix, and SLC35D1 may participate in CS biosynthesis.[60,61]

Cell Signaling Pathways and Growth Plate Maturation

Signaling pathways implicated by GWAS include PTH, PTHrP, IL6, Wnt signaling through association with FRZB, NCDN, TBC1D22A, and XIRP2.

Type 1 and 2 PTH/PTHrP receptor (PTH1R and PTH2R) belong to a family of G-protein-coupled receptors with 7 membrane-spanning helices.[62–64] PTH1R is expressed in bone and prehypertrophic chondrocytes and mediates mineral homeostasis.[62,65,66] Parathyroid hormone and parathyroid hormone–related peptide signaling were previously implicated in OA and skeletal homeostasis.[67] PTHrP regulates endochondral ossification during bone development and mice null for PTHrP expression show accelerated differentiation of chondrocytes in growing long bones.[68] PTH stimulates proliferation of prechondrocytes and inhibits collagen and matrix synthesis, regulating cartilage growth and chondrocyte apoptosis.[69] PTHrP acts as a local factor to regulate chondrogenesis and attenuating chondrocyte hypertrophy.[64,70] PTHrP is a central factor in the regulation of bone growth. Although the role of PTH1R and PTH2R in OCD is not currently known, a decrease in expression levels corresponding to an increase in OA severity has been reported in human subchondral osteoblasts.[71] Osteoblasts may be responsible for the initiation of OCD and OA, indicated by in vitro studies using a co-culture system comprising osteoarthritic osteoblasts and normal cartilage explants, in which cartilage degradation was initiated by enzymes produced by the osteoblasts.[72] Although PTH1R levels decrease, the levels of PTHrP have been shown to increase with increased OA severity.[73] PTH1R levels in chondrocytes have been evaluated in a rabbit model system over time.[74]

PTH1R was identified as a candidate gene for both equine and swine osteochondrosis,[27,34] whereas the related *PTH2R* was identified by Lampe and colleagues.[31] PTH1R is activated by PTH and PTHrP, both of which have been shown to regulate bone metabolism and differentiation.[70,75,76] PTHrP interacts with Indian hedgehog (IHH) and TGF-β to create a feedback loop that regulates the terminal differentiation of chondrocytes to hypertrophic cells.[8] Without PTHrP, chondrocytes prematurely differentiate into hypertrophic cells. PTH1R is vital for the appropriate signaling by PTHrP in the correct cells for differentiation of chondrocytes.[70] Previous experimentation by Semevolos and colleagues[76] found that PTHrP was upregulated in equine osteochondrosis by in situ hybridization and immunohistochemistry; however, PCR testing was inconclusive. A mutation associated with *PTH1R* can change the binding affinity of PTH and PTHrP, in turn, affecting the PTHrP, IHH, and TGF-β feedback loop essential for chondrocyte differentiation.

NCDN located on human chromosome 1.p34.3, encodes a leucine-rich cytoplasmic protein that functions as a negative regulator of calcium/calmodulin-dependent protein kinase II phosphorylation (CaMKII).[77] *NCDN* is expressed by chondrocytes, osteoblasts, and osteocytes within the skeleton, and evidence suggests that NCDN may be involved in bone metabolism.[78] Both the Wnt and PTHrP signaling pathways regulate CaMKII activity to support normal growth plate development, regulating the proliferative potential of chondrocytes.[79]

Cartilage (*CART1; ALX1*), located on human chromosome 12q21.31, encodes a homeobox transcription factor that plays a role in chondrocyte differentiation.[80,81] Gene variants of *FRZB* have been previously associated with OA.[82] *FRZB* encodes the secreted frizzled-related protein 3, which is a soluble inhibitor of the Wnt signaling pathway. Wnt signaling activity is increased in patients with OA.[83–85]

TBC1D22A, located on human chromosome 22q13.31, encodes a GTPase-activating protein. *XIRP2*, located on chromosome 2q24.3, encodes a cytosolic protein that interacts with actin stress fibers and protects actin filaments from depolymerization[86] in the cells of the myotendinous junction of skeletal muscle, among other locations. Inorganic phosphate transporter 1 (*PIT1;SLC20A1*), located on human chromosome 2q13, encodes a sodium-phosphate symporter that plays a role in phosphate transport in osteoblasts[87] and cartilage calcification.[88]

Galectin-3 (lectin, galactoside-binding soluble, 3 [*LGALS3*]), located on human chromosome 14q22.3, encodes an extracellular matrix protein that binds specifically to β-galactosides. Galectin-3 also can be found located in the nucleus and the cytoplasm of mature and early hypertrophic chondrocytes. Galectin plays an important role in skeletal development and in extracellular matrix assembly. Galectin-3 plays a role in the coordination between chondrocyte differentiation, hypertrophy, and subsequent vascular invasion essential for bone formation. In the absence of galectin-3, vascular invasion of hypertrophic cartilage is reduced.[89]

Calcitonin gene–related peptide-receptor component protein (*RCP9; CRCP*), located on human chromosome 7q11.21, encodes a membrane protein that functions as part of a receptor complex for a small neuropeptide that increases intracellular cAMP levels.[90]

Apart from *COL24A1* and *PTH1R*, no other specific genes were identified by more than one study; however, the collagen family was implicated in multiple studies. Many other genes have been identified inconsistently. One possible reason for the large number of QTLs identified may be the variation in breeds tested. Heritability varies by breed; the variability may be explained by different polymorphisms found in different breeds. *PTH1R* is a strong candidate gene for OCD, identified in both horses and pigs. Research on OCD and osteochondrosis has been completed in other animals, including dog and rat; however, genetic studies have not yet been completed.

Mitochondrial trans-2-enoyl CoA reductase (*MECR*), located on human chromosome 1p35.3, encodes a mitochondrial enzyme. Although it is not clear what role *MECR* might play in the onset and progression of OCD, metabolic factors play a role in osteochondrosis.[91] One significant marker region was shared by Orr and colleagues[24] and Teyssedre and colleagues[23] on chromosome 3 at 105 cM; however, neither article suggested genes of interest in this region. A BLAST search was completed for genes in the region, revealing leucine aminopeptidase 3 (*LAP3*) as a possible gene of interest in that region. Although no evidence currently supports a role for *LAP3* in OCD, future studies may provide this information.

SUMMARY

Although progress has been made, much about the genetic basis of OCD remains unknown. To understand OCD susceptibility genes, additional genetic analysis must be carried out in an unbiased fashion. GWAS provide this approach. Although accuracy and density of genotyping information may represent a limitation in the effort to match genotype with phenotype for OCD, continuing technical advances, coupled with decreasing costs of genome analysis, hold promise for the utilization of whole-genome DNA and RNA sequencing for patients. This review summarizes GWAS to date, and highlights the strength of genome-based approaches that use high-throughput methods in the search for causes and potential therapeutic targets for the treatment of OCD. Results from GWAS tend to cluster into thematic groups (**Fig. 2**).

A common theme within the genes identified by GWAS reviewed here include secreted proteins of the extracellular matrix and the genes encoding proteins that mediate vesicular transport, posttranslational modification, and safe passage through the cellular secretory pathway. A second theme that emerges is that of cell-signaling pathways known to regulate cellular differentiation for cells that play a critical role in growth plate development and maturation. Two pathways directly implicated are the PTH/PTHrP (by the identification of *PTH1R* and *PTH2R*) and Wnt (by the identification of *FRZB*) signaling pathways, both essential regulators of growth plate development. Established links exist between the gene clusters (see **Fig. 2**), because growth factors and cytokines regulate cellular responses that in turn lead to increases or decreases in the expression level and secretion of cell and tissue type-specific genes. The intersection of gene groups emerging from these studies may serve to guide future studies in OCD.

Much work has been done to understand OCD and osteochondrosis in humans and in animals, and an initial understanding of the etiology of this disease is forming. GWAS provide an unbiased approach for the identification of contributing genes. Horses have been investigated in several genetic studies, which often have included larger subject populations than studies performed in pigs. Swine research did not focus solely on osteochondrosis, but included other phenotypic traits relating to leg weakness. Additionally, many more SNPs were analyzed in horse studies compared with swine studies. Future studies are anticipated in equines, swine, and humans.

Although similarities exist between human OCD and osteochondrosis in the equine and swine systems, comparison of the results of equine and swine studies with OCD in humans must be based on similarities between these conditions. Osteochondrosis in

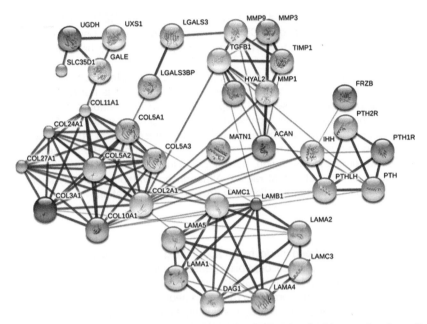

Fig. 2. STRING interaction network. *Search Tool for the Retrieval of Interacting Genes/Proteins* (STRING) is a database of known and predicted protein interactions. The interactions include direct (physical) and indirect (functional) associations. STRING quantitatively integrates interaction data. The database currently covers 5,214,234 proteins from 1133 organisms.[103] The interaction network was generated by seeding with genes identified through GWAS (Table 3). Additional interacting proteins were identified through STRINGS and are included in the network as likely candidates for contributing roles in OCD. Blue lines connecting each node are weighted for confidence of interaction, based on peer-reviewed, published information. More data exist to support an interaction between those nodes connected by the heavier blue lines. Genes cluster into (1) a collagen cluster, (2) a laminin cluster, (3) a cell-signaling cluster, (4) a matrix turnover cluster, and (5) a posttranslational modification cluster. Each of these clusters is linked by multiple connections.

humans is different from OCD in humans. However, improved disease definitions, as well as classification and comparison criteria, would advance the study of OCD irrespective of species. OCD is a multifactorial disease, eluding researchers due in part to low levels of statistical power and inconsistent results from study to study. GWAS stand to improve both the statistical power and consistency from study to study.

Differences in DNA methylation may be involved in the pathogenesis of OCD and must be analyzed in future studies. Subchondral bone homeostasis is perturbed in OCD, suggesting an interruption in the cyclic and sequential proliferation and differentiation of osteoclast and osteoblast precursor cells required for normal bone remodeling and growth. Methylation of cytosines in CpG-rich regions of DNA influence gene transcription and cell differentiation in the osteoblast lineage and osteoblast-osteocyte transition,[92,93] as shown by genome-wide methylation profiling of bone tissue in patients with osteoporosis and OA.[94] Future studies should include genome-wide methylation profiling for OCD to identify regions of differential methylation and to understand the relationship between methylation and gene expression in OCD. This approach has been successful in the analysis of osteoporosis and for OA, as DNA methylation represents an epigenetic level of regulation, methylation of

Table 3
Genes identified from genome-wide association studies used to seed the Search Tool for the Retrieval of Interacting Genes/Proteins (STRING) network (see Fig. 2)

●	LAMB1	Laminin, beta 1: Binding to cells via a high-affinity receptor, laminin is thought to mediate the attachment, migration and organization of cells into tissues during embryonic development by interacting with other extracellular matrix components. (1786 aa)
●	SLC35D1	Solute carrier family 35 (UDP-glucuronic acid/UDP-N-acetylgalactosamine dual transporter), member D1: Transports both UDP-glucuronic acid (UDP-GlcA) and UDP-N-acetylgalactosamine (UDP-GalNAc) from the cytoplasm to into the endoplasmic reticulum lumen. Participates in glucuronidation and/or chondroitin sulfate biosynthesis. (355 aa)
●	COL10A1	Collagen, type X, alpha 1: Type X collagen is a product of hypertrophic chondrocytes and has been localized to presumptive mineralization zones of hyaline cartilage. (680 aa)
●	LGALS3	Lectin, galactoside-binding, soluble, 3: Mediates with the alpha-3, beta-1 integrin the stimulation by CSPG4 of endothelial cells migration. Together with DMBT1, required for terminal differentiation of columnar epithelial cells during early embryogenesis. (250 aa)
●	ACAN	Aggrecan: This proteoglycan is a major component of extracellular matrix of cartilaginous tissues. A major function of this protein is to resist compression in cartilage. It binds avidly to hyaluronic acid via an N-terminal globular region. (2416 aa)
●	PTH2R	Parathyroid hormone 2 receptor: This is a specific receptor for parathyroid hormone. The activity of this receptor is mediated by G proteins that activate adenylyl cyclase. PTH2R may be responsible for PTH effects in a number of physiologic systems. (550 aa)
●	FRZB	Frizzled-related protein: Soluble frizzled-related proteins (sFRPS) function as modulators of Wnt signaling through direct interaction with Wnts. They have a role in regulating cell growth and differentiation in specific cell types. SFRP3/FRZB is involved in limb skeletogenesis. Antagonist of Wnt8 signaling. Regulates chondrocyte maturation and long bone development. (325 aa)
●	MMP3	Matrix metallopeptidase 3 (stromelysin 1, progelatinase): Can degrade fibronectin; laminins; gelatins of type I, III, IV, and V; collagens III, IV, X, and IX, and cartilage proteoglycans. Activates procollagenase. (477 aa)
●	COL3A1	Collagen, type III, alpha 1: Collagen type III occurs in most soft connective tissues along with type I collagen. (1466 aa)
●	UGDH	UDP-glucose dehydrogenase: Biosynthesis of glycosaminoglycans; hyaluronan, chondroitin sulfate, and heparan sulfate. (494 aa)
●	PTH1R	Parathyroid hormone 1 receptor: This is a receptor for parathyroid hormone and for parathyroid hormone-related peptide. The activity of this receptor is mediated by G proteins that activate adenylyl cyclase and also a phosphatidylinositol-calcium second messenger system. (593 aa)
●	COL27A1	Collagen, type XXVII, alpha 1: Plays a role during the calcification of cartilage and the transition of cartilage to bone (1860 aa)
●	HYAL2	Hyaluronoglucosaminidase 2: Hydrolyzes high molecular weight hyaluronic acid to produce an intermediate-sized product that is further hydrolyzed by sperm hyaluronidase to give small oligosaccharides. Associates with and negatively regulates MST1R. (473 aa)
●	COL24A1	Collagen, type XXIV, alpha 1: Participates in regulating type I collagen fibrillogenesis during fetal development. (1714 aa)

(continued on next page)

Table 3 (continued)		
●	COL5A1	Collagen, type V, alpha 1: Type V collagen is a member of group I collagen (fibrillar forming collagen). It is a minor connective tissue component of nearly ubiquitous distribution. Type V collagen binds to heparan sulfate, thrombospondin, heparin, and insulin. (1838 aa)
●	MATN1	Matrilin 1, cartilage matrix protein: A major component of the extracellular matrix of cartilage. It binds to collagen. (496 aa)
●	COL5A2	Collagen, type V, alpha 2: Type V collagen is a member of group I collagen (fibrillar-forming collagen). It is a minor connective tissue component of nearly ubiquitous distribution. Type V collagen binds to heparan sulfate, thrombospondin, heparin, and insulin. Type V collagen is a key determinant in the assembly of tissue-specific matrices. (1499 aa)

Genes identified and reviewed were input into the STRING network. All genes included in the STRING network and a description of the genes are included.

CpG-rich sequences of the promoter regions represses genes known to play roles in bone formation and bone resorption. Epigenetic mechanisms modulate the expression of proteases and other cartilage constituents, recently reviewed by Reynard and Loughlin[95] and Barter and colleagues.[96] However, little is known about the role of methylation in pathogenesis of osteochondral changes in OCD. Unlike the genome, epigenetic markers may be transmitted unmodified through cell division or, alternatively, change with the cell environment and stresses to the skeletal system. Age-related changes in DNA methylation patterns may provide information regarding the age of onset for OCD. Further studies are required to identify the mechanisms involved.

Small noncoding microRNAs (miRNAs) are important regulators of coordinated gene expression[97] and must be included in future studies. miRNAs act by forming base pairs with their complementary messenger RNA molecules, usually in the 3′-untranslated region of specific genes to silence gene expression.[98] miRNAs have been shown to be necessary for normal skeletal development[99] and may also play a role during disease progression. For example, miR-140 was shown to be expressed only in cartilaginous tissues,[100] and in its absence, miR-140$^{(-/-)}$ mice manifested a mild skeletal phenotype with a short stature. miR-140$^{(-/-)}$ mice experienced proteoglycan loss and fibrillation of articular cartilage.[101]

Studies in humans will not only identify possible genes that cause OCD, but will also validate the work done in other species. McCoy and colleagues[102] recently highlighted the similarities between osteochondrosis in animals and OCD in humans, including histological appearance of end-stage lesions, radiographic/MRI changes, clinical presentation, and predilection sites, strengthening the case for common pathogenesis. Additional studies will help to discover the role that secretion of extracellular matrix proteins, such as COL24A1, and signaling pathways, such as the ones mediated by PTH1R, play in the onset and progression of OCD. Further use of genomic and molecular analysis techniques, including GWAS, comprehensive genomic analysis of DNA methylation patterns, and analysis of miR expression to collect information from multiple species will improve our understanding of the pathogenesis of OCD, and identify molecular targets for the development of targeted preventions of joint damage and progression to OA. Future work should use the strengths of high-efficiency methods that are becoming increasingly available to understand the molecular mechanisms underlying OCD and the link between the protein secretion pathway and cell-signaling pathways that regulate chondrocyte and osteoblast differentiation during growth plate maturation.

ACKNOWLEDGMENTS

The authors acknowledge the technical assistance of Barbara Jibben. Research reported in this publication was supported by an Institutional Development Award (IDeA) from the National Center for Research Resources and the National Institute of General Medical Sciences of the National Institutes of Health under grant numbers P20 RR016454 and P20 GM103408, the Boise State University Student Research Initiative Program, and the Department of Biologic Sciences (BIOL451).

REFERENCES

1. Edmonds E, Shea K. Osteochondritis dissecans: editorial comment. Clin Orthop Relat Res 2013;471:1105–6.
2. Lykkjen S, Dolvik N, McCue M, et al. Genome-wide association analysis of osteochondrosis of the tibiotarsal joint in Norwegian standardbred trotters. Anim Genet 2010;2(Suppl 41):111–20.
3. König F. The classic: on loose bodies in the joint. 1887. Clin Orthop Relat Res 2013;471:1107–15.
4. Shea K, Jacobs J Jr, Carey J, et al. Osteochondritis dissecans knee histology studies have variable findings and theories of etiology. Clin Orthop Relat Res 2013;471:1127–36.
5. Edmonds E, Polousky J. A review of knowledge in osteochondritis disse-cans:123 years of minimal evolution from König to the ROCK study group. Clin Orthop Relat Res 2013;471:1118–26.
6. Thacker M, Dabney K, Mackenzie W. Osteochondritis dissecans of the talar-head: natural history and review of literature. J Pediatr Orthop B 2012;21: 373–6.
7. Polousky J. Juvenile osteochondritis dissecans. Sports Med Arthrosc 2011;19: 56–63.
8. Ytrehus B, Carlson C, Ekman S. Etiology and pathogenesis of osteochondrosis. Vet Pathol 2007;44:429–48.
9. Kocher M, Tucker R, Ganley T, et al. Management of osteochondritis dissecans of the knee: current concepts review. Am J Sports Med 2006;34:1181–91.
10. Cahill B. Osteochondritis dissecans of the knee: treatment of juvenile and adult forms. J Am Acad Orthop Surg 1995;3:237–47.
11. Stattin E, Tegner Y, Domellof M, et al. Familial osteochondritis dissecans associated with early osteoarthritis and disproportionate short stature. Osteoarthritis Cartilage 2008;16:890–6.
12. Lindén B, Telhag H. Osteochondritis dissecans. A histologic and autoradiographic study in man. Acta Orthop Scand 1977;48:682–6.
13. Twyman R, Desai K, Aichroth P. Osteochondritis dissecans of the knee. A long-term study. J Bone Joint Surg Br 1991;73:461–4.
14. Chambers H, Shea K, Anderson A, et al. Diagnosis and treatment of osteochondritis dissecans. J Am Acad Orthop Surg 2011;19:297–306.
15. McIlwraith C. Inferences from referred clinical cases of osteochondritis dissecans. Equine Veterinary Journal 1993;25(S16):2042–3306.
16. Jorgensen B, Arnbjerg J, Aaslyng M. Pathological and radiological investigations on osteochondrosis in pigs, associated with leg weakness. Zentralbl Veterinarmed 1995;42:489–504.
17. Laenoi W, Uddin J, Cinar M, et al. Quantitative trait loci analysis for leg weakness-related traits in a duroc X pietrain crossbred population. Genet Sel Evol 2011;43:13.

18. Jeffcott L. Osteochondrosis in the horse—searching for the key to pathogenesis. Equine Vet J 1991;23:331–8.

19. Stattin E, Wiklund F, Lindblom K, et al. A missense mutation in the aggrecan C-type lectin domain disrupts extracellular matrix interactions and causes dominant familial osteochondritis dissecans. Am J Hum Genet 2010;86:126–37.

20. Mubarak S, Carroll N. Familial osteochondritis dissecans of the knee. Clin Orthop Relat Res 1979;140:131–6.

21. Wittwer C, Lohring K, Drogemuller C, et al. Mapping quantitative trait loci for osteochondrosis in fetlock and hock joints and palmar/plantar osseus fragments in fetlock joints of South German coldblood horses. Anim Genet 2007;38:350–7.

22. Wittwer C, Hamann H, Rosenberger E, et al. Genetic parameters for the prevalence of osteochondrosis in the limb joints of South German coldblood horses. J Anim Breed Genet 2007;124:302–7.

23. Teyssedre S, Dupuis M, Guerin G, et al. Genome-wide association studies for osteochondrosis in French trotter horses. J Anim Sci 2012;90:45–53.

24. Orr N, Hill E, Gu J, et al. Genome-wide association study of osteochondrosis in the tarsocrural joint of Dutch warmblood horses identifies susceptibility loci on chromosomes 3 and 10. Anim Genet 2012;44(4):408–12. http://dx.doi.org/10.1111/age.12016.

25. Wittwer C, Hamann H, Distl O. The candidate gene Xirp2 at a quantitative gene locus on equine chromosome 18 associated with osteochondrosis in fetlock and hock joints of South German coldblood horses. J Hered 2009;100:481–6.

26. Corbin L, Blott S, Swinburne J, et al. A genome-wide association study of osteochondritis dissecans in the Thoroughbred. Mamm Genome 2012;23:294–303.

27. Dierks C, Lohring K, Lampe V, et al. Genome-wide search for markers associated with osteochondrosis in Hanoverian warmblood horses. Mamm Genome 2007;18:739–47.

28. Dierks C, Komm K, Lampe V, et al. Fine mapping of a quantitative trait locus for osteochondrosis on horse chromosome 2. Anim Genet 2010;41:87–90.

29. Lampe V, Dierks C, Distl O. Refinement of a quantitative trait locus on equine chromosome 5 responsible for fetlock osteochondrosis in Hanoverian warmblood horses. Anim Genet 2009;40:553–5.

30. Lampe V, Dierks C, Komm K, et al. Identification of a new quantitative trait locus on equine chromosome 18 responsible for osteochondrosis in Hanoverian warmblood horses. J Anim Sci 2009;87:3477–81.

31. Lampe V, Dierks C, Distl O. Refinement of a quantitative gene locus on equine chromosome 16 responsible for osteochondrosis in Hanoverian warmblood horses. Animal 2009;3:1224–31.

32. Wittwer C, Dierks C, Hamann H, et al. Associations between candidate gene markers at a quantitative trait locus on equine chromosome 4 responsible for osteochondrosis dissecans in fetlock joints of South German coldblood horses. J Hered 2008;99:125–9.

33. Laenoi W, Rangkasenee N, Uddin M, et al. Association and expression study of MMP3, TGF beta 1 and Col10a1 as candidate genes for leg weakness-related traits in pigs. Mol Biol Rep 2012;39:3893–901.

34. Andersson-Eklund L, Uhlhorn H, Lundeheim N, et al. Mapping quantitative trait loci for principal components of bone measurements and osteochondrosis scores in a WildBoar X large white intercross. Genet Res 2000;75:223–30.

35. Fairbank H. Osteochondritis dissecans. Br J Surg 1933;21:67–82.

36. Laor T, Zbojniewicz A, Eismann E, et al. Juvenile osteochondritis dissecans: is it a growth disturbance of the secondary physis of the epiphysis? AJR Am J Roentgenol 2012;199:1121–8.
37. Chiroff R, Cooke C 3rd. Osteochondritis dissecans: a histologic and microradiographic analysis of surgically excised lesions. J Trauma 1975;15:689–96.
38. Csóka A, Scherer S, Stern R. Expression analysis of six paralogous human hyaluronidase genes clustered on chromosomes 3p21 and 7q31. Genomics 1999;15:356–61.
39. Csoka A, Frost G, Stern R. The six hyaluronidase-like genes in the human and mouse genomes. Matrix Biol 2001;20:499–508.
40. Flannery C, Little C, Hughes C, et al. Expression and activity of articular cartilage hyaluronidases. Biochem Biophys Res Commun 1998;251:824–9.
41. Chow G, Knudson W. Characterization of promoter elements of the human HYAL-2 gene. J Biol Chem 2005;280:26904–12.
42. Deak F, Wagener R, Kiss I, et al. The matrilins: a novel family of oligomeric extracellular matrix proteins. Matrix Biology 1999;18:55–64.
43. Chapman K, Mortier G, Chapman K, et al. Mutations in the region encoding the von Willebrand factor A domain of matrilin-3 are associated with multiple epiphyseal dysplasia. Nature Genetics 2001;28:393–6.
44. Mostert A, Dijkstra P, Jansen B, et al. Familial multiple epiphyseal dysplasia due to a matrilin-3 mutation: further delineation of the phenotype including 40 years follow-up. American Journal of Medical Genetics 2003;120:490–7.
45. Makitie O, Mortier G, Czarny-Ratajczak M, et al. Clinical and radiographic findings in multiple epiphyseal dysplasia caused by MATN3 mutations: description of 12 patients. American Journal of Medical Genetics 2004;125:278–84.
46. Mabuchi A, Haga N, Maeda K, et al. Novel and recurrent mutations clustered in the von Willebrand factor A domain of MATN3 in multiple epiphyseal dysplasia. Human Mutation 2004;24:439–40.
47. Borochowitz Z, Scheffer D, Adir V, et al. Spondylo-epi-metaphyseal dysplasi (SEMD) matrilin 3 type: homozygote matrilin 3mutation in a novel form of SEMD. Journal of Medical Genetics 2004;41:366–72.
48. Stefansson S, Jonsson H, Ingvarsson T, et al. Genomewide scan for hand osteoarthritis: a novel mutation in matrilin-3. American Journal of Human Genetics 2003;72:1448–59.
49. Pullig O, Weseloh G, Klatt A, et al. Matrilin-3 in human articular cartilage: increased expression in osteoarthritis. Osteoarthritis and Cartilage 2002;10:253–63.
50. Min J, Meulenbelt I, Riyazi N. Association of matrilin-3 polymorphisms with spinal disc degeneration and osteoarthritis of the first carpometacarpal joint of the hand. Annals of the Rheumatic Diseases 2006;65:1060–6.
51. Pullig O, Tagariello A, Schweizer A, et al. MATN3 (matrilin-3) sequence variation (pT303M) is a risk factor for osteoarthritis of the CMC1 joint of the hand, but not for knee osteoarthritis. Annals of the Rheumatic Diseases 2007;66:279–80.
52. Koch M, Laub F, Zhou P, et al. Collagen XXIV, a vertebrate fibrillar collagen with structural features of invertebrate collagens: selective expression in developing cornea and bone. J Biol Chem 2003;278:43236–44.
53. Skagen P, Horn T, Kruse H, et al. Osteochondritis dissecans (OCD), an endoplasmic reticulum storage disease?: a morphological and molecular study of OCD fragments. Scand J Med Sci Sports 2011;21:e17–33.

54. Matsuo N, Tanaka S, Yoshioka H, et al. Collagen XXIV (Col24a1) gene expression is a specific marker of osteoblast differentiation and bone formation. Connect Tissue Res 2008;49:68–75.

55. Wang W, Olson D, Liang G, et al. Collagen XXIV (Col24α1) promotes osteoblastic differentiation and mineralization through TGF-β/Smads signaling pathway. Int J Biol Sci 2012;8:1310–22.

56. Suleman F, Gualeni B, Gregson H, et al. A novel form of chondrocyte stress is triggered by a COMP mutation causing pseudoachondroplasia. Hum Mutat 2012;33:218–31.

57. Nundlall S, Rajpar M, Bell P, et al. An unfolded protein response is the initial cellular response to the expression of mutant matrilin-3 in a mouse model of multiple epiphyseal dysplasia. Cell Stress Chaperones 2010;15:835–49.

58. Zhu Y, Han S, Zhao H, et al. Comparative analysis of serum proteomes of degenerative scoliosis. J Orthop Res 2011;29:1896–903.

59. Huan C, Greene K, Shui B, et al. mCLCA4 ER processing and secretion requires luminal sorting motifs. Am J Physiol Cell Physiol 2008;295:C279–87.

60. Muraoka M, Kawakita M, Ishida N. Molecular characterization of human UDP-glucuronic acid/UDP-N-acetylgalactosamine transporter, a novel nucleotide sugar transporter with dual substrate specificity. FEBS Lett 2001;495:87–93.

61. Hiraoka S, Furuichi T, Nishimura G, et al. Nucleotide-sugar transporter SLC35D1 is critical to chondroitin sulfate synthesis in cartilage and skeletal development in mouse and human. Nat Med 2007;13:1363–7.

62. Mannstadt M, Juppner H, Gardella T. Receptors for PTH and PTHrP: their biological importance and functional properties. Am J Physiol 1999;277:F665–75.

63. Abou-Samra A, Uneno S, Jueppner H, et al. Non-homologous sequences of parathyroid hormone and the parathyroid hormone related peptide bind to a common receptor on ROS 17/2.8 cells. Endocrinology 1989;125:2215–7.

64. Amizuka N, Henderson J, White J, et al. Recent studies on the biological action of parathyroid hormone (PTH)-related peptide (PTHrP) and PTH/PTHrP receptor in cartilage and bone. Histol Histopathol 2000;15:957–70.

65. Lee K, Deeds J, Segre G. Expression of parathyroid hormone-related peptide and its receptor messenger ribonucleic acids during fetal development of rats. Endocrinology 1995;136:453–63.

66. Lee K, Lanske B, Karaplis A, et al. Parathyroid hormone-related peptide delays terminal differentiation of chondrocytes during endochondral bone development. Endocrinology 1996;137:5109–18.

67. Elliott K, Chapman K, Day-Williams A, et al. Evaluation of the genetic overlap between osteoarthritis with body mass index and height using genome-wide association scan data. Ann Rheum Dis 2013;72:935–41.

68. Lanske B, Karaplis A, Lee K, et al. PTH/PTHrP receptor in early development and Indian hedgehog-regulated bone growth. Science 1996;273:663–6.

69. Harrington E, Lunsford L, Svoboda K. Chondrocyte terminal differentiation, apoptosis, and type X collagen expression are downregulated by parathyroid hormone. Anat Rec A Discov Mol Cell Evol Biol 2004;281:1286–95.

70. Vortkamp A, Lee K, Lanske B, et al. Regulation of rate of cartilage differentiation by Indian hedgehog and PTH-related protein. Science 1996;273:613–22.

71. Hilal G, Massicotte F, Martel-Pelletier J, et al. Endogenous prostaglandin E2 and insulin-like growth factor 1 can modulate the levels of parathyroid hormone receptor in human osteoarthritic osteoblasts. J Bone Miner Res 2001;16:713–21.

72. Westacott C, Webb G, Warnock M, et al. Alteration of cartilage metabolism by cells from osteoarthritic bone. Arthritis Rheum 1997;40:1282–91.

73. Kohno H, Shigeno C, Kasai R, et al. Synovial fluids from patients with osteoarthritis and rheumatoid arthritis contain high levels of parathyroid hormone-related peptide. J Bone Miner Res 1997;12:847–54.

74. Becher C, Szuwart T, Ronstedt P, et al. Decrease in the expression of the type 1 PTH/PTHrP receptor (PTH1R) on chondrocytes in animals with osteoarthritis. Journal of Orthopaedic Surgery and Research 2010;5:28.

75. Kulkarni N, Halladay D, Miles R, et al. Effects of parathyroid hormone on wnt signaling pathway in bone. J Cell Biochem 2005;95:1178–90.

76. Semevolos S, Brower-Toland B, Bent S, et al. Parathyroid hormone-related peptide and Indian hedgehog expression patterns in naturally acquired equine osteochondrosis. J Orthop Res 2002;20:1290–7.

77. Dateki M, Horii T, Kasuya Y, et al. Neurochondrin negatively regulates CaMKII phosphorylation, and nervous system-specific gene disruption results inepileptic seizure. J Biol Chem 2005;280:20503–8.

78. Ishiduka Y, Mochizuki R, Yanai K, et al. Induction of hydroxyapatite resorptive activity in bone marrow cell populations resistant to bafilomycin A1 by a factor with restricted expression to bone and brain, neurochondrin. Biochim Biophys Acta 1999;1450:92–8.

79. Li Y, Ahrens M, Wu A, et al. Calcium/calmodulin-dependent protein kinase II activity regulates the proliferative potential of growth plate chondrocytes. Development 2011;138:359–70.

80. Zhai L, Zhao K, Wang Z, et al. Mesenchymal stem cells display different gene expression profiles compared to hyaline and elastic chondrocytes. Int J Clin Exp Med 2011;4:81–90.

81. Thompson H, Griffiths J, Jeffery G, et al. The retinal pigment epithelium of the eye regulates the development of scleral cartilage. Dev Biol 2010;347:40–52.

82. Baker-Lepain J, Lynch J, Parimi N, et al. Variant alleles of the WNT antagonist FRZB are determinants of hip shape and modify the relationship between hip shape and osteoarthritis. Arthritis Rheum 2012;64:1457–65.

83. Velasco J, Zarrabeitia M, Prieto J, et al. Wnt pathway genes in osteoporosis and osteoarthritis: differential expression and genetic association study. Osteoporos Int 2010;21:109–18.

84. Luyten F, Tylzanowski P, Lories R. Wnt signaling and osteoarthritis. Bone 2009; 44:522–7.

85. Corr M. Wnt-beta-catenin signaling in the pathogenesis of osteoarthritis. Nat Clin Pract Rheumatol 2008;4:550–6.

86. Pacholsky D, Vakeel P, Himmel M, et al. Xin repeats define a novel actin-binding motif. J Cell Sci 2004;117:5257–68.

87. Caverzasio J, Bonjour J. Characteristics and regulation of Pi transport in osteogenic cells for bone metabolism. Kidney Int 1996;49:975–80.

88. Sugita A, Kawai S, Hayashibara T, et al. Cellular ATP synthesis mediated by type III sodium-dependent phosphate transporter Pit-1 is critical to chondrogenesis. J Biol Chem 2011;286:3094–103.

89. Colnot C, Sidhu S, Balmain N, et al. Uncoupling of chondrocyte death and vascular invasion in mouse galectin 3 null mutant bones. Dev Biol 2001;229:203–14.

90. Uezono Y, Bradley J, Min C, et al. Receptors that couple to 2 classes of G proteins increase cAMP and activate CFTR expressed in *Xenopus* oocytes. Receptors Channels 1993;1:233–41.

91. Sarneveld A, van Weeren PR. Conclusions regarding the influence of exercise on the development of the equine musculoskeletal system with special reference to osteochondrosis. Equine Vet J Suppl 1999;31:112–9.

92. Delgado-Calle J, Sanudo C, Bolado A, et al. DNA methylation contributes to the regulation of sclerostin expression in human osteocytes. J BoneMiner Res 2012; 27:926–37.

93. Delgado-Calle J, Sanudo C, Fernandez A, et al. Role of DNA methylation in the regulation of the RANKL-OPG system in human bone. Epigenetics 2012;7:83–91.

94. Delgado-Calle J, Fernández A, Sainz J, et al. Genome-wide profiling of bone reveals differentially methylated regions in osteoporosis and osteoarthritis. Arthritis Rheum 2013;65:197–205.

95. Reynard L, Loughlin J. Genetics and epigenetics of osteoarthritis. Maturitas 2012;71:200–4.

96. Barter M, Bui C, Young D. Epigenetic mechanisms in cartilage and osteoarthritis: DNA methylation, histone modifications and microRNAs. Osteoarthritis Cartilage 2012;20:339–49.

97. Chiang H, Schoenfeld L, Ruby J, et al. Mammalian microRNAs: experimental evaluation of novel and previously annotated genes. Genes Dev 2010;24: 992–1009.

98. Mendell J. MicroRNAs: critical regulators of development, cellular physiology and malignancy. Cell Cycle 2005;4:1179–84.

99. Kapinas K, Delany A. MicroRNA biogenesis and regulation of bone remodeling. Arthritis Res Ther 2011;13:220.

100. Miyaki S, Sato T, Inoue A, et al. MicroRNA-140 plays dual roles in both cartilage development and homeostasis. Genes Dev 2010;24:1173–85.

101. Miyaki S, Asahara H. Macro view of microRNA function in osteoarthritis. Nat Rev Rheumatol 2012;8:543–52.

102. McCoy AM, Toth F, Dolvik NI, et al. Articular osteochondrosis: a comparison of naturally-occurring human and animal disease. Osteoarthritis and Cartilage 2013;21(11):1638–47. http://dx.doi.org/10.1016/j.joca.2013.08.011.

103. Franceschini A, Szklarczyk D, Frankild S, et al. STRING v9.1: protein-protein interaction networks, with increased coverage and integration. Nucleic Acids Res 2013;41(Database issue):D808–15.

Imaging of Osteochondritis Dissecans

Andrew M. Zbojniewicz, MD*, Tal Laor, MD

KEYWORDS

- Osteochondritis dissecans • Cartilage • Ossification variation
- Magnetic resonance imaging (MRI) • Radiography • Knee • Elbow • Ankle

KEY POINTS

- Osteochondritis dissecans (OCD) can affect both adults and children, however the imaging characteristics and significance of imaging findings can differ in the juvenile subset with open physes.
- Radiography and magnetic resonance imaging (MRI) are the primary modalities used to aid in diagnosis, to define a treatment plan, to monitor progress, to assess surgical intervention, and to identify postoperative complications.
- Newer imaging techniques under continuous development may improve the accuracy of MRI for diagnosis and staging of OCD, and eventually may help to predict the durability of tissue-engineered constructs and cartilage repair.

Osteochondritis dissecans (OCD) can affect both adults and children, but the juvenile subset that is present in patients with open physes may have a different clinical course and prognosis.[1–5] The appearance and significance of imaging findings has similarly been shown to be different in children compared with adults.[6,7]

Radiographs constitute the initial imaging evaluation of patients with OCD but also are used to evaluate for lesion healing. Magnetic resonance imaging (MRI) may be used to confirm diagnosis and to aid in treatment planning. MRI also is useful to monitor healing with conservative management or after surgical intervention, and to aid in identification of complications in patients with continued pain.

KNEE
Imaging Diagnosis of OCD

The American Academy of Orthopaedic Surgeons (AAOS) guidelines for diagnosis and treatment of OCD give a weak recommendation for the use of conventional radiographs in patients with knee symptoms and/or signs suggesting OCD, based on a lack of strong evidence to suggest their efficacy.[8] However, radiographs are

Disclosures: The authors have no disclosures.
Department of Radiology, Cincinnati Children's Hospital Medical Center, University of Cincinnati College of Medicine, 3333 Burnet Avenue, Cincinnati, OH 45229, USA
* Corresponding author.
E-mail address: andrew.zbojniewicz@cchmc.org

inexpensive and readily available and therefore remain the mainstay of both diagnosis and monitoring of patients with OCD. Despite their continued widespread use, radiographs are limited by the lack of visualization of unossified elements, the inability to assess for mechanical instability, and the use of ionizing radiation.

Radiographic examination of the knee in the setting of possible OCD typically includes anteroposterior (AP), lateral, tunnel, and Merchant or sunrise views. The tunnel view is typically obtained with a posterior-to-anterior (PA) beam direction and approximately 30° to 40° of knee flexion, allowing improved visualization of the posterior femoral condyles. The Merchant view is performed with the patient supine and the knee flexed approximately 30° to best depict the femoral trochlea and patellar articular surface. OCD of the knee most commonly involves the lateral aspect of the medial femoral condyle (69%), followed by the lateral femoral condyle (15%), the patella (5%), and the femoral trochlea (1%).[9] The characteristic appearance of an OCD lesion on radiographs consists of a well-circumscribed lucent defect in subchondral bone that may or may not contain internal bone density (**Figs. 1** and **2**). However, in young children, subchondral irregularity or lucencies of either or both femoral condyles may reflect normal development, often referred to as irregular ossification or developmental ossification variation.

Similar to their recommendation regarding the use of radiography for diagnosis, the AAOS clinical practice guideline summary for diagnosis and treatment of OCD gave a weak recommendation for the use of MRI to characterize a known OCD lesion previously diagnosed with radiographs or to aid with diagnosis of concomitant disorder.[8] This weak recommendation was chosen in part because, at the time the guidelines were developed, no study had addressed the additional value of the use of MRI in the setting of an OCD lesion diagnosed with radiography. In addition, they cited inconsistent correlation of the MRI appearance of lesion instability with arthroscopic findings. In current practice, MRI is frequently used to attempt differentiation of a

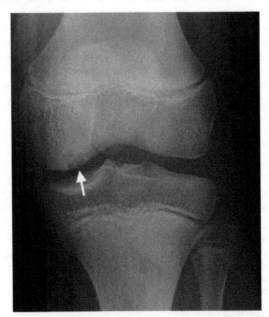

Fig. 1. Juvenile OCD. AP standing radiograph from an 11-year-old boy football player shows a poorly circumscribed lucency (*arrow*) in the lateral aspect of the medial femoral condyle.

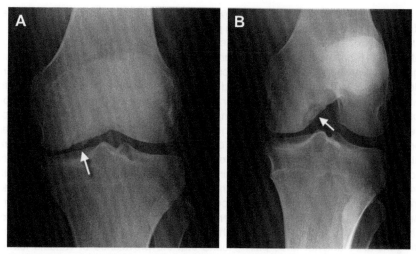

Fig. 2. Skeletally mature patient with OCD. (*A*) AP standing radiograph in a 17-year-old boy shows a well-circumscribed fragment of bone (*arrow*) within a lucent defect of the lateral aspect of the medial femoral condyle. (*B*) PA tunnel view, flipped to correspond with part (*A*), again shows the bone fragment (*arrow*).

developmental ossification variation from OCD, and following diagnosis of OCD to guide treatment by the assessment of whether a lesion is likely to be stable at the time of arthroscopy.

Developmental Ossification Variation and Juvenile Osteochondritis Dissecans of the Distal Femur

Sontag and Pyle[10] in 1941 followed by Caffey and colleagues[11] in 1958 found that distal femoral epiphyseal irregularities are common in children (aged 1–13 years) and resolve spontaneously, but can appear similar to radiographic findings in children diagnosed with OCD. Since that time, the differentiation of ossification variation from osteochondritis dissecans in children continues to be a difficult and controversial area of inquiry, with most attempts at delineation focused on MRI features.

An initial attempt to characterize ossification variations of the posterolateral femoral condyle on MRI was a report of 4 boys, aged 8 to 11 years, who despite osseous irregularity on MRI lacked clinical symptoms of the knee.[12] The investigators described these sites as islets of accessory ossification similar in signal intensity to the subchondral bone. The adjacent lucent zones identified on accompanying radiographs corresponded with areas similar in signal intensity to cartilage on MRI. Because earlier reports depicted juvenile OCD as abnormalities with hyperintense signal separating a lesion from the adjacent cartilage, the investigators concluded that, "MR imaging of osteochondritis dissecans may be clearly differentiated from those anomalies of ossification."

However, differentiation between the two diagnoses is not always well defined. Gebarski and Hernandez[13] suggested that accessory ossification centers and spiculations of the posterior inferocentral femoral condyles in children with substantial unossified epiphyseal cartilage, intact overlying cartilage, no associated edema, and bicondylar or bilateral location likely represent normal variants of ossification. A puzzle-piece configuration of the bone in the absence of edema is likely also a normal variation.[13] However, central intracondylar lesions with adjacent edema were findings associated with OCD.[13] The investigators concluded that normal ossification variation can mimic early stage OCD, and this overlap in appearance might explain the great difference in outcomes associated with juvenile and adult forms of OCD.

Jans and colleagues[14] used these previously described criteria in their study population of 315 patients to divide children into a group with ossification variation and a group with juvenile OCD, in order to confirm previously described criteria and provide additional MRI features that might distinguish these two entities. They concluded that ossification variability did not occur in girls more than 10 years of age or in boys more than 13 years of age, was not seen if the child had 10% or less of residual unossified epiphyseal cartilage, and was found in the posterior third with occasional extension to the middle third of either femoral condyle. In contrast, OCD was rare in children with greater than 30% of residual unossified epiphyseal cartilage and was most frequently seen in the medial middle third of the femoral condyle. Extension into the intracondylar region was associated with OCD. It was also suggested that ossification variation extended deeper into the adjacent bone and showed no perilesional edema, whereas OCD lesions tended to be flatter and accompanied by adjacent bone marrow edema pattern.[14] Another study from the same group that did not exclude patients with general or anterior knee pain[15] found that the prevalence of variable femoral condylar ossification decreases with age, and is most common in boys. Peak age ranges for ossification variation was 2 to 12 years in boys and 2 to 10 years in girls. The same group in a third study concluded that ossification variations are not more common in children with OCD, and do not evolve into OCD lesions.[16]

In addition, it has been reported that juvenile OCD lesions consistently show disruption of the overlying normal thin hyperintense hemispherical secondary physis responsible for epiphyseal growth on water-weighted MRI sequences.[7] There may also be increased width of the unossified epiphyseal cartilage overlying OCD lesions compared with the adjacent, unaffected portions of condyle.[7] Whether the secondary physis is always continuous and the epiphyseal cartilage is similar in width to adjacent portions of the condyles in children with normal ossification variation is yet to be determined. **Table 1** summarizes many of the demographic and MRI features that have been reported with normal developmental ossification variation and with juvenile OCD that may be useful in their differentiation (**Figs. 3** and **4**).

Table 1
Features that may differentiate developmental ossification variation and juvenile OCD

Ossification Variation	Juvenile OCD
Demographics	
Girls <10 y of age, boys <13 y of age	Girls or boys >8 y of age
MRI Features	
No adjacent bone marrow edema	Adjacent bone marrow edema
Posterior third location ± extension to middle third; not anterior third	Usually middle third location
No intracondylar extension	—
Spiculation, puzzle pieces, accessory ossification centers	—
>10% residual cartilage	Rare with >30% residual cartilage
Deeper lesion (lesional angle <105°)	Flatter lesion (lesional angle >105°)
—	Disruption of secondary physis
—	Widened overlying unossified epiphyseal cartilage

Data from Refs.[7,13–16]

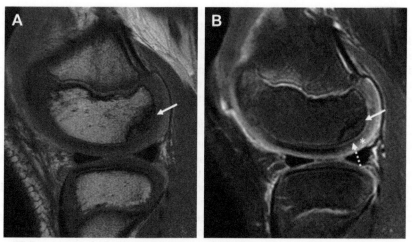

Fig. 3. Normal ossification variation. (*A*) Sagittal proton density–weighted image and (*B*) fat-suppressed T2-weighted image of the lateral femoral condyle from a 10-year-old boy show a puzzle-piece configuration (*arrows*) within the posterior third of the lateral femoral condyle. There is no adjacent bone marrow edema pattern, the secondary physis (*dashed arrow* in *B*) is intact, and the overlying unossified epiphyseal cartilage (*asterisk* in *B*) is not widened.

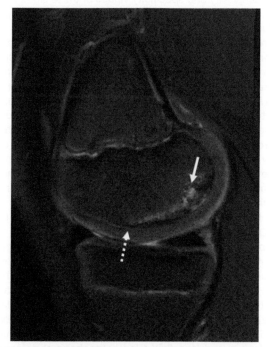

Fig. 4. Juvenile OCD. Sagittal fat-suppressed T2-weighted image of the medial femoral condyle from an 11-year-old boy shows osseous irregularity involving the middle and posterior thirds of the medial femoral condyle. There is adjacent bone marrow edema pattern (*arrow*) and the secondary physis (*dashed arrow*) becomes discontinuous at the lesion.

To date, although these studies have provided practitioners with useful guidelines to aid with differentiation of these two entities, the ability to define distinguishing features on MRI between normal ossification variation and juvenile OCD is limited by the retrospective nature of imaging reports, the absence of surgical and pathologic correlation, and the lack of longitudinal follow-up in children. However, correlation of clinical symptoms such as knee pain and swelling with the MRI appearance and patient demographics is often adequate to distinguish between these two entities.

Lesion Characteristics and Treatment Planning

Because of the inherent limitations of radiographic evaluation, which include underestimation of lesion size and inability to assess the integrity of overlying cartilage, MRI often is used to aid with formulation of a treatment plan.[9] Typical MRI sequences performed for the evaluation of OCD lesions include intermediate-weighted or T2-weighted fast spin echo (FSE) sequences in the sagittal or coronal plane with at least one plane fat suppressed, as well as a three-dimensional (3D) T1-weighted gradient recalled echo (GRE) sequence with fat suppression, typically in the sagittal plane.

There is abundant literature regarding the usefulness of MRI for staging OCD and the assessment of lesion stability.[6,17–25] De Smet and colleagues[17] in 1990 first reported one of the most widely recognized systems for the assessment of OCD lesion stability in the knee and ankle. The investigators identify 4 signs on T2-weighted images that were associated with instability of an OCD lesion, namely (1) hyperintense signal at the fragment-femur interface, (2) adjacent focal cystic areas, (3) displaced fragments within the joint, and (4) defects in articular cartilage. In 1996, the group went on to publish sensitivity and specificity values of these signs with slightly refined MRI criteria to include (1) either a well-defined or ill-defined line of hyperintense signal equal to that of fluid at the fragment-bone interface that measures 5 mm or more in length, (2) a discrete round focus of hyperintense signal deep to the OCD lesion measuring 5 mm or more, (3) a focal defect in the overlying articular cartilage that measures more than 5 mm in width, and (4) hyperintense signal equal to that of fluid that traverses both the articular cartilage and subchondral bone and extends into the lesion (**Figs. 5** and **6**).[18] Using these criteria, De Smet and colleagues[18] found a sensitivity of 97% and specificity of 100% for the detection of unstable OCD lesions. However, the investigators recognized that their patient cohort was small and therefore accurate conclusions regarding the value of imaging in the determination of lesion stability were limited. They suggested that, although a hyperintense T2 signal line present at the fragment-bone interface was sensitive, it may be less specific and may not necessarily indicate instability. In contrast, the investigators found that their other three signs were 100% specific for instability.

De Smet and colleagues[17,18] criteria did not distinguish between juvenile and adult patients with OCD, and the youngest patient in their cohort was 13 years old. To address this limitation, subsequent work by Kijowski and colleagues[6] determined that the aforementioned MRI criteria for lesion instability had a high specificity in adults, but not in children with OCD. This report used variations of the original criteria described in 1990, which included (1) linear rim of hyperintense signal surrounding the OCD on T2-weighted images with no mention of its need to be similar to signal intensity of joint fluid, (2) cysts surrounding the OCD lesion with no mention of cyst size, (3) hyperintense T2 signal fracture line that extends through the articular cartilage that overlies the OCD lesion, and (4) a fluid-filled osteochondral defect with no mention of size. These criteria were 100% sensitive and 100% specific for adult OCD, but although they were 100% sensitive for juvenile OCD, they were only 11% specific. The findings indicate that a hyperintense T2 signal rim or cystlike focus does not

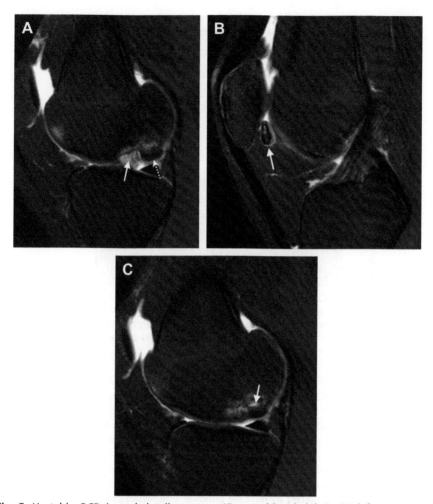

Fig. 5. Unstable OCD in a skeletally mature 15-year-old girl. (*A*) Sagittal fat-suppressed T2-weighted image of the lateral aspect of the medial femoral condyle shows a focal defect in articular cartilage anteriorly (*arrow*) that measures more than 5 mm. An in situ fragment (*dashed arrow*) is seen within the posterior portion of the OCD. (*B*) The displaced osteochondral fragment (*arrow*) from the anterior portion of the lesion is seen in a more midline image. (*C*) There is a hyperintense T2 signal line 6 mm in length equal to the signal intensity of fluid at the lesion fragment-bone interface (*arrow*), which in addition to the incongruity of the articular surface indicates instability.

necessarily indicate instability in juvenile OCD (**Fig. 7**). However, if there was hyperintense rimlike T2 signal equal to that of joint fluid at the fragment-bone interface with a second deeper linear margin of hypointense T2 signal (**Fig. 8**), in addition to multiple sites of discontinuity of subchondral bone, these findings combined had both 100% sensitivity and 100% specificity for the determination of juvenile OCD instability. In addition, multiple cystlike foci or a single cystlike focus grater than 5 mm had sensitivities ranging from 25% to 38%, but specificity of 100% for the detection of instability (**Fig. 9**). A summary of imaging criteria used to suggest instability in both adult and juvenile OCD is provided in **Table 2** .

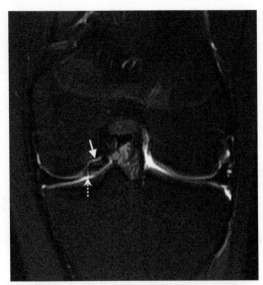

Fig. 6. Unstable OCD. Coronal fat-suppressed T2-weighted image in a different skeletally immature 15-year-old girl shows a vertical hyperintense T2 signal line (*dashed arrow*) that traverses articular cartilage and courses toward the OCD fragment-bone interface. A more horizontal hyperintense T2 signal line (*arrow*) equal to fluid continues between the fragment and the underlying bone.

More recent studies[20,24] regarding the usefulness of MRI in the determination of juvenile OCD lesion stability corroborated these findings and revealed high sensitivity and low specificity for De Smet and colleagues'[17,18] original criteria.

However, these studies also did not use the refined criteria for juvenile OCD presented by Kijowski and colleagues[6] to assess for degree of improvement from the original criteria.

Lesion size measurement on MRI has been reported to be useful for treatment planning in children with a stable juvenile OCD lesion. Wall and colleagues[5] reported that lesion dimension normalized to femoral condyle size when plotted on a nomogram could be used to predict patient outcome. A recent study by Krause and colleagues[26] similarly suggested that age along with findings on MRI were able to help guide the choice between conservative and surgical treatment. A nomogram based on age, normalized lesion width, and size of cystlike foci on MRI was able to determine the healing potential of an OCD lesion at 6 months, and a cystlike focus smaller than 1.3 mm was associated with healing by 12 months.[26]

Posttreatment Imaging: Expected Findings and Complications

Following the diagnosis of an OCD lesion, a patient undergoes either conservative or surgical treatment. Conservative treatment of a stable juvenile OCD lesion may consist of activity modification, cast immobilization, or bracing and typically ranges in duration from 3 to 12 months.[9] Surgical treatment usually is used following failed conservative treatment or in the setting of an unstable OCD lesion, and entails either a primary repair or a salvage procedure.[9] Primary repair includes transarticular or retroarticular drilling and stabilization procedures, with or without bone grafting, or debridement of the lesion.[9] Salvage procedures include microfracture, osteochondral autograft or allograft, and autologous chondrocyte implantation (ACI).[9]

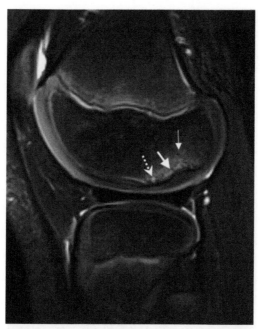

Fig. 7. Stable juvenile OCD. Sagittal fat-suppressed T2-weighted image from a 12-year-old shows a moderately hyperintense T2 signal rim (*thicker arrow*), but the hyperintense signal is not equal to fluid and does not contain an adjacent linear margin of hypointense T2 signal. There is a bone marrow edema pattern (*thinner arrow*), and a single small (<6 mm) cyst (*dashed arrow*) at the anterior margin of the lesion. The patient also has a discoid lateral meniscus. The OCD lesion was determined to be stable at surgery 1 month later.

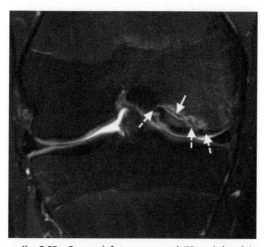

Fig. 8. Unstable juvenile OCD. Coronal fat-suppressed T2-weighted image in a skeletally immature 17-year-old boy shows a rim of hyperintense T2 signal equal to fluid signal, with a deeper linear hypointense T2 signal margin (*solid arrow*), and multiple breaks in subchondral bone (*dashed arrows*).

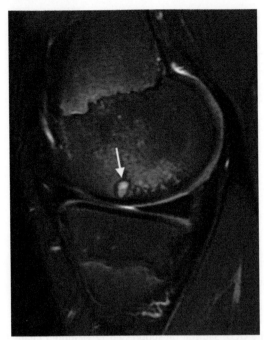

Fig. 9. Large cystlike focus. Sagittal fat-suppressed T2-weighted image from a 14-year-old skeletally immature boy shows a single large 6-mm hyperintense signal cystlike focus (*arrow*) associated with a juvenile OCD lesion, which at arthroscopy was found to be unstable.

Table 2
MRI findings that suggest unstable OCD

Adult OCD[18] (T2-weighted Images)		Juvenile OCD[6] (T2-weighted Images)	
Well-defined or ill-defined hyperintense signal line equal to fluid signal at fragment-bone interface ≥5 mm	97% specificity, 100% sensitivity	Rimlike hyperintense signal equal to joint fluid signal + second deeper linear margin of low signal + multiple sites of discontinuity of subchondral bone	100% sensitive, 100% specific
Discrete round focus of high signal intensity ≥5 mm		Multiple cystlike foci or single cystlike focus >5 mm	Sensitivity 25%–38%, specificity 100%
Focal defect in articular cartilage >5 mm in width		—	—
Hyperintense signal line equal to fluid signal that traverses both articular cartilage and subchondral bone		—	—

Radiographs are the most frequent imaging modality used for monitoring children who undergo a conservative treatment plan. Assessment of healing on radiographs seems straightforward, but this can be deceiving. A variety of terms are used in the literature to describe radiographic signs of healing of an OCD lesion, and, as such, there are no standardized criteria. Terms such as reossification, disappearance of the radiolucent zone, resolution of the sclerotic rim, radiographic union of the lesion, resolution of the lesion, and resolution of the radiolucent demarcation around the lesion have all been used to indicate radiographic healing (**Fig. 10**).[27] A recent study by Parikh and colleagues[27] that did not use standardized criteria questions the reliability of the determination of healing based on conventional radiographs. Four reviewers evaluated radiographs from 39 children (mean age of 11.9 years) with OCD lesions of the knee who had been treated conservatively for 6 months. There was poor interrater reliability for the determination of healing of knee OCD lesions on

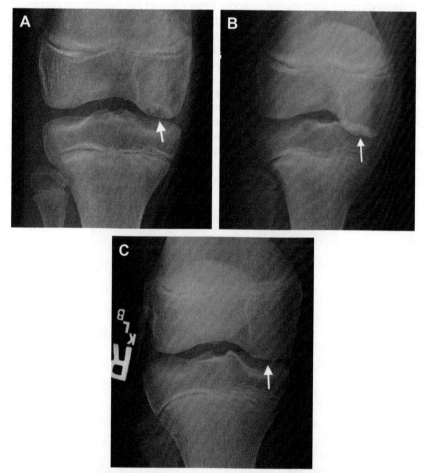

Fig. 10. Juvenile OCD lesion in an 11-year-old girl gymnast that healed over time with conservative management. (*A*) AP radiograph shows a well-circumscribed lucent defect (*arrow*) in the central medial femoral condyle. (*B*) Approximately 4 months later, there is increased sclerosis (*arrow*) within the OCD lesion. (*C*) Approximately 23 months after (*A*), the lesion appears healed (*arrow*).

radiographs, which suggests that standardized criteria are needed.[27] In addition, variation in image acquisition between patient visits can result in substantial difference in interpretation of healing over time. Tunnel views, in particular, can show different parts of the femoral condyles based on how steeply the radiography tube is angled and on the extent of knee flexion.

Radiographic findings that indicate previous surgical treatment commonly include transarticular screws (**Fig. 11**) and retroarticular drill tracks. Indicators of healing following surgery are similar to those recognized in the nonoperated knee, such as bone formation within the OCD defect and loss of the radiolucent zone of demarcation about the lesion. However, visualization of the condylar surface can be obstructed by screws.

MRI is often performed to assess healing in patients being treated conservatively, as well as in those who have undergone surgery. The recommended time interval for the assessment of healing on MRI in patients who undergo conservative management is variable depending on institutional protocol (time allowed for healing by conservative management) and surgeon preference. Although the recent study by Krause and colleagues[26] used MRI examinations exclusively at 6 months and 12 months to document healing, at our institution serial radiographs are used primarily for the first 6 months, with MRI reserved for cases with indeterminate healing, obtained usually at 6 months. MRI findings that suggest healing following conservative management include interval decrease or resolution in surrounding bone marrow edema pattern, decrease in lesion size, decrease or resolution of the hyperintense T2 signal rim or cystlike foci, and ingrowth of bone within the bed of the OCD lesion with bridging to the adjacent subchondral bone, best seen on non–fat-suppressed T1-weighted or GRE-weighted images.

Following surgical treatment of OCD, MRI allows a noninvasive assessment of repair tissue at both the articular surface and the bone-cartilage interface.[28] In order to evaluate repair cartilage in OCD lesions, MRI sequences similar to those used for the

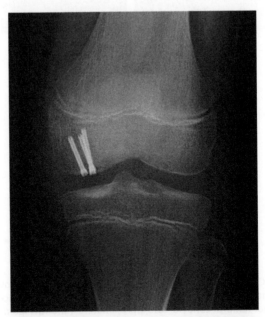

Fig. 11. AP radiograph from a 9-year-old boy shows internal fixation of a juvenile OCD lesion of the medial femoral condyle by 3 headless compression screws.

diagnosis of OCD and those recommended by the International Cartilage Reparative Society for use in the evaluation of native cartilage, namely intermediate-weighted or T2-weighted FSE with or without fat suppression and T1-weighted GRE with fat suppression, should be used.[28] Non–fat-suppressed techniques result in greater signal to noise, which allows improved visualization of small abnormalities within cartilage. Therefore, protocols should include at least one plane without fat suppression to evaluate cartilage and one plane with fat suppression because of its increased sensitivity for marrow signal abnormalities. A T1-weighted sequence that is sensitive for marrow fat signal should also be performed in either the coronal or sagittal plane in order to assess for osseous integration. If MRI evaluation following a salvage procedure is desired, an initial examination at 3 to 6 months after surgery to assess the volume and integration of tissue is suggested,[28] followed by an additional examination at least 1 year after the procedure to assess incorporation and to identify postoperative complications.[28]

Retroarticular drilling and bone grafting does not result in the breach of articular cartilage. Therefore, lesional healing is expected to have a similar appearance to that observed with conservative management, namely the resolution of the bone marrow edema pattern and the hyperintense T2 signal rim or cystlike foci, as well as osseous ingrowth or incorporation of bone graft that fills the bed of the OCD lesion (**Fig. 12**). Surgical procedures that include microfracture and subchondral drilling frequently are used to allow multipotential stem cells in the surrounding marrow access into the OCD site and/or into areas of articular cartilage loss. The goal of these procedures is to promote healing of the OCD lesion or stimulate fibrocartilaginous tissue repair. Microfracture typically is used for cartilage defects smaller than 2 to 4 cm^2.[29]

Following microfracture, it can take up to 2 years for the defect to fill in completely with smooth and well-defined margins (**Fig. 13**).[28] In the first few months (usually 3–6 months) following the microfracture procedure, only thin and indistinct repair tissue may be present and should not be interpreted as treatment failure.[28] Because of a less organized matrix with increased water mobility, early reparative fibrocartilage may also show hyperintense signal on T2-weighted or intermediate-weighted FSE images compared with the hypointense signal intensity of adjacent native cartilage.[28] With maturation, this reparative tissue decreases in signal intensity and eventually may even become hypointense relative to native cartilage.[28,30] Although a subchondral bone marrow edema pattern may be present normally after surgery, it is expected to decrease over time.[28] A persistent bone marrow edema pattern in subchondral bone and lack of filling of the defect over time indicates treatment failure.[28] In contrast, overgrowth of subchondral bone is commonly seen (25%–49% of patients) and may not adversely affect clinical outcomes.[28,30] However, in select patients in whom bone overgrowth allows only a thin layer of reparative cartilage and poor lesional filling, there may be less favorable functional outcomes.[30] In addition, fissures are commonly seen at the junction of reparative fibrocartilage and native cartilage, but are not necessarily clinically relevant.[30]

Following a salvage procedure with osteochondral autograft, the defect should be filled by the graft. Eventual integration is heralded by trabecular incorporation between the plug and native bone, with uniform fat signal intensity on T1-weighted images (**Fig. 14**).[28,30] Small fissures between cartilage associated with the plug and the adjacent native cartilage often persist despite the graft otherwise appearing well incorporated.[28] These fissures have been shown at second-look arthroscopy to be filled with a fibrocartilaginous bond formed by organized scar tissue, and should not necessarily raise concern.[30] There should be a smooth transition between the surface of the native and the graft cartilage with complete restoration of the normal radius of curvature of

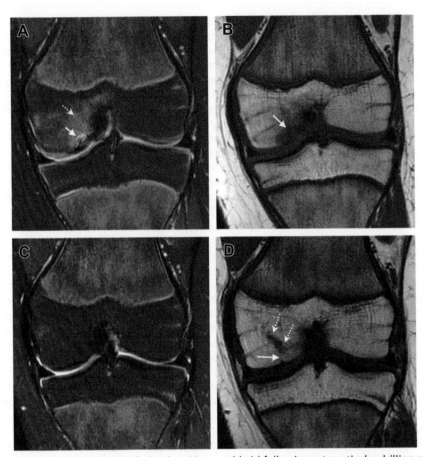

Fig. 12. Healed juvenile OCD lesion in a 14-year-old girl following retroarticular drilling and bone graft placement. (*A*) Coronal fat-suppressed T2-weighted image shows a hyperintense T2 signal rim (*arrow*) and bone marrow edema pattern (*dashed arrow*) within the medial femoral condyle. (*B*) The OCD lesion and adjacent bone marrow edema pattern are hypointense on this coronal T1-weighted image (*arrow*). (*C*) Approximately 14 months following surgery, a coronal fat-suppressed T2-weighted image shows resolution of the edema pattern and hyperintense signal rim. (*D*) Coronal T1-weighted image from the same time as (*C*) shows ingrowth of bone (*arrow*) at the site of the OCD lesion and adjacent retroarticular drill tracts (*dashed arrows*).

the condylar surface, which helps to maintain the biomechanical integrity of the plug.[28] Bone marrow edema pattern in and about the graft may be present in the first year following the procedure, but gradual reduction in this finding over time is expected.[28] Edema pattern in the graft has been reported in a small number of cases as late as 3 years following the procedure.[28] Joint effusion and synovial hypertrophy can persist for up to 2 years, and alone do not indicate graft failure.[28]

Lack of incorporation of an osteochondral autograft is suggested by fluid signal intensity at the interface between the graft and native bone, cystlike foci within subchondral bone, and a persistent bone marrow edema pattern (**Fig. 15**). Incongruity of the articular surface resulting in a loss of the normal radius of curvature can follow technical problems related to the initial press-fit placement of the graft or can be a more

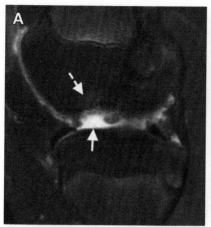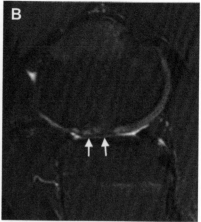

Fig. 13. Microfracture surgery. (*A*) Sagittal fat-suppressed T2-weighted image shows a large defect in articular cartilage (*arrow*) and subchondral bone marrow edema pattern (*dashed arrow*), consistent with an unstable juvenile OCD lesion. (*B*) Approximately 14 months following microfracture surgery, there is excellent fill of the OCD defect by reparative fibro-cartilage, which has a similar signal intensity to native cartilage, and a smooth contour to the articular surface (*arrows*).

delayed manifestation of graft degradation of subsidence.[30] Another postsurgical complication is osteonecrosis of the plug, which is suggested on MRI by graft resorption and failure of osseous integration.[28]

Similar to osteochondral autografts, osteochondral allografts should be assessed for degree of fill of the osteochondral defect, integration of the graft, and a smooth transition between the surface of the native cartilage and the graft cartilage. Likewise, bone marrow edema pattern may be seen within the graft in the first 3 to 6 months following surgery, with a gradual decrease expected over time. Persistent bone marrow edema pattern 12 months after surgery, fluid signal intensity at the graft-host interface, or surface collapse may be indicators of graft rejection or lack of incorporation.[28] In addition, low signal intensity within the graft on all pulse sequences may be related to loss of bone viability and eventual implant failure.[30]

More recently, synthetic biphasic copolymer plugs have been used as a scaffold for bone and cartilage growth both to backfill donor sites in the setting of osteochondral autograft harvest or for primary cartilage repair.[30] Unlike autologous bone plugs, these are a scaffold and as such, presence of depression of the plug without restoration of the radius of curvature, resorption at the interface with native bone, and incomplete fill at less than 12 months all can be normal findings.[30] Complete incorporation can take more than 2 years, so a diagnosis of incomplete incorporation should be applied with caution.[30]

As opposed to microfracture, which is used for small lesions, ACI is often used for large defects (>2 cm^2) in articular cartilage. The classic procedure consists of a 2-stage operation; one to harvest healthy chondrocytes to be cultured in vitro for 3 to 5 weeks, and a second to implant the cultured chondrocytes with coverage by a periosteal flap that is secured in place with fibrin glue or sutures.[28] A second-generation procedure uses a bilayer collagen membrane instead of the periosteal flap.[28] A third-generation procedure, also known as matrix-induced autologous chondrocyte implantation (MACI) uses a collagen bilayer membrane as well, but with chondrocytes seeded into the membrane, allowing precise sizing of the membrane and fixation with fibrin glue alone. For deeper lesions (>8–10 mm), bone grafting is often

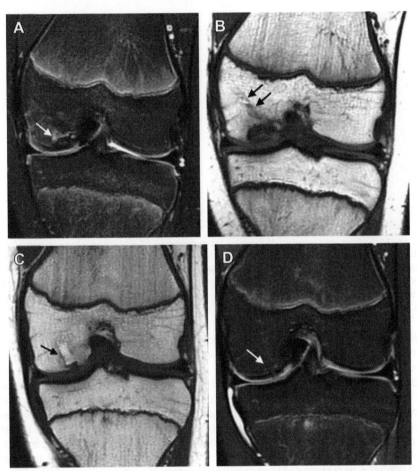

Fig. 14. Osteochondral autograft. (*A*) Coronal fat-suppressed T2-weighted image shows an OCD lesion (*arrow*) of the medial femoral condyle. (*B*) Coronal T1-weighted image shows tracks (*black arrows*) from retroarticular drilling and bone grafting performed approximately 1 year previously. (*C*) Coronal T1-weighted image obtained approximately 1 year after salvage procedure with placement of an osteochondral autograft shows excellent healing with incorporation of the osteochondral plug to the surrounding bone (*arrow*). (*D*) There is resolution of the hyperintense signal rim (*arrow*) on the coronal fat-suppressed T2-weighted image.

performed in conjunction with ACI. This is either performed as a staged operation with a separate surgery for bone grafting, or more recently with a "sandwich" technique. This technique consists of application of cancellous bone graft deep within the bed of the defect followed by placement of cultured chondrocytes "sandwiched" between periosteal or bilayer collagen membranes or by using two bilayer collagen membranes seeded with chondrocytes (MACI membranes).[28,31]

Three phases have been described in association with healing following ACI. The proliferative phase refers to the initial 6 weeks following surgery when the soft, primitive repair tissue begins to fill the site, although complete fill has been seen as early as 3 weeks after the procedure.[30] The transition phase involves expansion of the extracellular matrix and results in a gelatinlike consistency that occurs after 7 weeks to

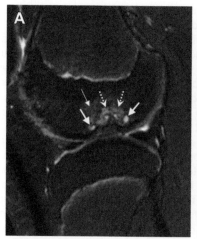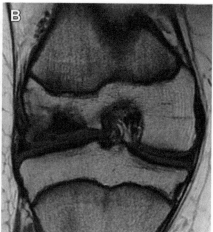

Fig. 15. Osteochondral autograft. (*A*) Sagittal fat-suppressed T2-weighted image shows hyperintense signal cystlike foci within subchondral bone (*thicker arrows*), and bone marrow edema pattern in the osteochondral plugs (*dashed arrows*) and in the surrounding bone (*thinner arrow*), which suggest lack of graft incorporation. (*B*) Coronal T1-weighted image shows hypointense signal at the OCD site, consistent with lack of osseous integration.

6 months, followed by the remodeling phase when hyalinelike repair cartilage is formed, at approximately 6 months to 3 years.[30] The MRI appearance reflects the histology, with early (less than 6 months after surgery) repair cartilage expected to be of hyperintense signal on T2-weighted or intermediate-weighted images relative to native cartilage, caused by the disorganization of the tissue architecture with resultant increased water content.[30] A gradual decrease in signal intensity is expected over time.[28,30] Filling of the defect by repair tissue can be described as flush, depressed, or proud, with a percent fill often characterized as either greater than or less than 50% of the depth of native cartilage.[28,30] Although ideally there should be complete filling of the defect with restoration of the normal radius of curvature of the articular surface, underfilling may not be clinically significant and requires further intervention in only approximately 2% of cases.[28,30] The interface of reparative cartilage with native cartilage is frequently not smooth, with small fissures less than 2 mm in width commonly seen.[30] In contrast, larger fissures are concerning for failed intergration.[30]

Two complications exclusive to ACI are cartilage delamination and cartilage overgrowth. Delamination typically occurs within 6 to 9 months of the procedure, is rare, and is seen in less than 5% of patients.[30] In situ delamination is indicated by fluid signal intensity between the cartilage repair tissue and the subchondral bone, whereas a displaced delaminated graft manifests as a fluid-filled defect at the repair site with a displaced intra-articular body.[30] Cartilage overgrowth typically occurs at 3 to 9 months after surgery and may consist of hypertrophy of the periosteal cover or thickening of the matrix.[30] On MRI, this is seen as extension of the periosteal cover or matrix beyond the normal contour of the articular cartilage or extension over the adjacent native cartilage.[30] Although frequently asymptomatic, patients can present with pain or a catching sensation that may require arthroscopic resection.[30] Persistence in subchondral bone marrow edema pattern over time and development of subchondral cysts also are concerning findings that may be seen with lack of integration.[30]

Transarticular screws or bioabsorbable pins often are used for fixation of an OCD lesion after primary repair, or occasionally as part of a salvage procedure. The severity of metallic screw artifact on MRI depends on the type of hardware used, typically stainless steel or titanium. Stainless steel screws can obscure much, if not all, of the operative site (**Fig. 16**), whereas titanium screws result in minimal artifact (**Fig. 17**). Imaging parameters that can reduce MRI artifact from metal include the use of an increased bandwidth, small field of view, high-resolution matrix, thin slices, shorter echo time, and avoidance of fat-suppression techniques. The use of a short tau inversion recovery sequence also can reduce metal artifact. As an alternative, a new 3D FSE metal reduction sequence is now available for use in routine clinical practice that allows improved visualization of soft tissues around metal implants.

Bioabsorbable pins do not produce artifact on MRI. A study on the imaging appearance of polydioxanone biodegradable pins found that pins are linear in configuration and nearly always hypointense on T1-weighted images throughout the time course following surgery, whereas on T2-weighted images they tend to change gradually from hypointense to hyperintense signal over the first 12 months following placement, possibly because of hydrolyzed debris or fluid (see **Fig. 17**B).[28,32] Bone marrow edema pattern around the pins is seen in a minority of cases, generally decreasing over time.[32] In the study by Sirlin and colleagues,[32] 80% of the pins completely resorbed by 2 years.

Complications associated with bioabsorbable pins include failure of fixation or fracture, with subsequent displacement of all or part of the pin into the joint (**Fig. 18**). Transarticular screws can back out slightly, becoming proud relative to the articular surface, which may result in cartilage abnormalities of the adjacent tibia (see **Fig. 17**B). Radiographs are inadequate to define the relationship of screws to the articular surface, because articular cartilage and, in the case of juvenile OCD, unossified

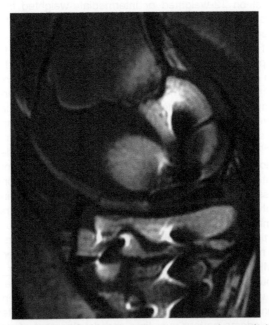

Fig. 16. Artifact from stainless steel compression screws in the medial femoral condyle. Sagittal fat-suppressed T2-weighted image shows substantial metallic artifact that results in poor fat suppression and nonvisualization of the area surrounding the screws and the articular surface. There is also artifact from additional hardware in the proximal tibia.

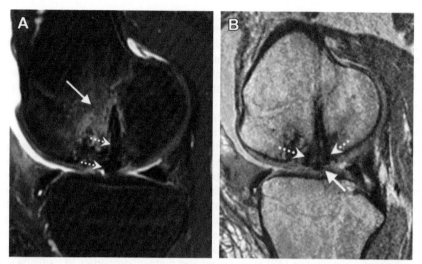

Fig. 17. Artifact from titanium compression screw in the lateral femoral condyle. (*A*) Sagittal fat-suppressed T2-weighted image shows only a small amount of artifact around the screw (*dashed arrows*). There is visualization of much of the OCD site as well adjacent bone marrow edema pattern (*solid arrow*). (*B*) Oblique sagittal 3D FSE proton density–weighted image in the same patient reformatted into the plane of the screw shows to better advantage the head of the screw (*arrow*). It has backed out slightly from the condyle and is in close approximation to the tibial articular surface. Bioabsorbable pins (*dashed arrows*) also are seen on either side of the compression screw.

epiphyseal cartilage cannot be visualized. However, MRI can be used to see the cartilage and evaluate the transarticular screws.

Future Developments in MRI of OCD

Recent developments in advanced imaging techniques may ultimately improve the accuracy of MRI in the diagnosis of OCD, may enable the refinement of treatment algorithms, and may further enhance the postsurgical assessment. One such imaging technique currently in clinical practice is a 3D FSE sequence capable of providing

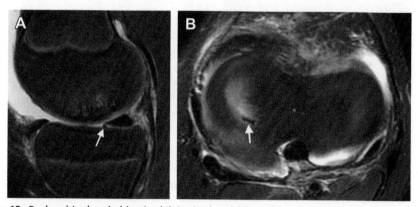

Fig. 18. Broken bioabsorbable pin. (*A*) Sagittal and (*B*) axial fat-suppressed T2-weighted images show a displaced screw fragment (*arrows*) lying inferior to the posterior horn of the medial meniscus.

high-resolution images with isotropic voxels. This technique allows thin sections (on the order of 1 mm or less) that can be reformatted into multiple planes with less volume averaging artifact, and already has been shown to increase the accuracy of MRI in the definition of abnormalities of articular cartilage in the knee.[33] This sequence may have a role in the improvement of accurate characterization of OCD lesions relative to arthroscopy and in the identification of complications following treatment (see **Fig. 17**B; **Fig. 19**).

Although most traditionally used MRI sequences subjectively evaluate the morphology of articular cartilage, newer techniques such as T2 mapping, T1ρ, and delayed gadolinium-enhanced MRI of cartilage (dGEMRIC) allow quantitative assessment of the composition of articular cartilage, as reflected by a tissue's T1 or T2 relaxation properties. These techniques give providers insight into the ultrastructure and biochemical properties of cartilage repair tissue and may allow objective measurement of treatment outcome, possibly even obviating biopsy, which traditionally has been the gold standard in the evaluation of success of repair (**Fig. 20**).[28,30,34] These quantitative sequences also have a potential role in the evaluation of unossified nonarticular cartilage in the setting of juvenile OCD. In addition, investigation is underway into the correlation between quantitative MRI assessment and material properties of cartilage with the hopes that imaging may eventually be able to predict the durability of tissue-engineered constructs and cartilage repair.[34]

ELBOW

OCD of the elbow most frequently involves the capitellum, although it also may involve the trochlea, radial head, and olecranon.[35] OCD needs to be differentiated from Panner disease, typically a self-limiting disorder of the capitellum that resolves with rest and little or no deformity. Panner disease is not associated with instability and as

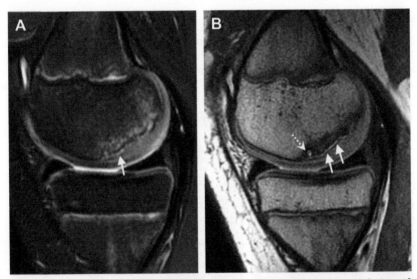

Fig. 19. (A) Sagittal fat-suppressed T2-weighted image shows a juvenile OCD lesion of the medial femoral condyle. There is a focal area of fluid signal intensity (*arrow*) at the interface between the OCD lesion and the subchondral bone. (B) Sagittal 3D FSE proton density–weighted image shows a well-defined hyperintense rim at the OCD-bone interface (*arrows*) and a small cystlike focus (*dashed arrow*) anteriorly.

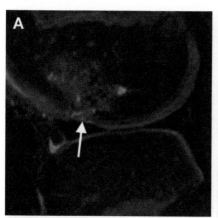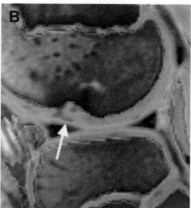

Fig. 20. T2 map of reparative cartilage. (*A*) Sagittal fat-suppressed T2-weighted image shows heterogeneous intermediate to hyperintense T2 signal material (*arrow*) within a site of microfracture performed 3 months earlier. This appearance suggests early reparative fibrocartilage. (*B*) Sagittal color-coded map of T2 relaxation time values shows abnormal red color (*arrow*) at the site of the reparative fibrocartilage, consistent with an abnormally long T2 relaxation time compared with the green color within the adjacent normal cartilage. The prolonged T2 relaxation time indicates disorganized tissue with greater mobility of water.

such only shows abnormal radiolucency, flattening or irregularity of the capitellum on radiographs, or hypointense T1 signal and possibly mild hyperintense T2 signal on MRI, but no loose bodies (**Fig. 21**). In contrast, OCD in the elbow has a limited capacity for healing with a potential for fragmentation and formation of loose intra-articular bodies, which occasionally result in degenerative joint disease. Panner disease is seen typically in young, growing children less than 10 years of age, whereas OCD usually presents in the young adolescent athlete with average age range of onset of 12 to 17 years.[35]

Radiographic examination in a patient suspected of having OCD of the elbow consists of an AP view in full extension and a lateral view with 90° of flexion. Radiographic findings of capitellar OCD include rarefaction/radiolucency, flattening of the articular surface, fragmentation with demarcating sclerosis, and intra-articular bodies.[35] Radial head enlargement and osteophyte production infrequently are seen as late findings.[35]

Staging was reportedly developed by Minami and colleagues, in which a grade 1 lesion was described as a translucent or cystic shadow of the middle or lateral aspect of the capitellum, a grade 2 lesion showed a split line or clear zone of demarcation between the lesion and subchondral bone, and a grade 3 lesion was characterized by an intra-articular loose body.[35] However, recent studies have questioned the sensitivity of radiographs for diagnosis and characterization of capitellar OCD.[36,37] Kijowski and De Smet[37] found that, even with a retrospective review, radiographs alone had limited sensitivity in detecting OCD of the capitellum and associated intra-articular loose bodies. In this study, which included 15 patients, only 66% of OCD were identified on initial interpretation of radiographs and only 57% of intra-articular bodies were seen. Because of the limitations in the standard AP and lateral elbow evaluation for diagnosis of OCD, it has been suggested by other investigators that adding an AP view with the elbow in 45° of flexion may improve radiographic detection of capitellar OCD.[35]

Because of limitations in radiographic evaluation, MRI frequently is performed in patients suspected of having capitellar OCD but who have normal radiographs, or in

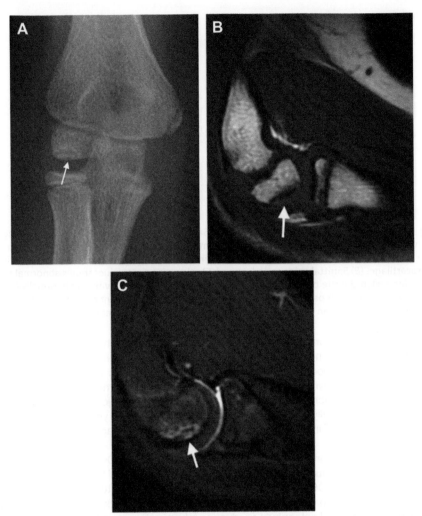

Fig. 21. Panner disease. (*A*) AP radiograph of an 8-year-old boy with elbow pain shows irregularity (*arrow*) of the capitellar ossification center. (*B*) Sagittal T1-weighted image shows hypointense signal (*arrow*) at the site of irregularity. (*C*) Fat-suppressed T2-weighted image shows mildly hyperintense signal (*arrow*) at the same location.

patients diagnosed with OCD who require further evaluation. Similar to MRI indications for OCD of the knee, the primary role of MRI for evaluating a known OCD of the elbow is to detect an unstable lesion, which will alter treatment planning and prognosis.

Kijowski and DeSmet[38] found that the criteria defined for OCD of the knee by DeSmet and colleagues[17,18] also can be applied to the assessment of lesion stability at the elbow (**Fig. 22**).

Jans and colleagues,[39] who used the conditions described by Kijowski and colleagues[6] for the assessment of instability of juvenile OCD in the knee, found that these criteria, when used together, were 100% sensitive for the assessment of instability of OCD lesions at the elbow in patients with a mean age of 14 years of age, although each

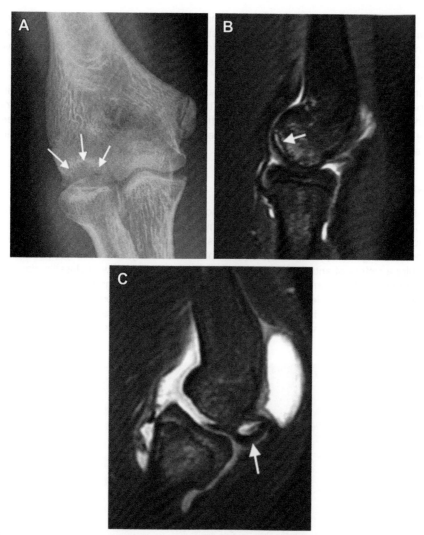

Fig. 22. Unstable capitellar OCD. (*A*) Frontal radiograph shows the characteristic focal lucency in the capitellum (*arrows*) indicating an OCD lesion. (*B*) Sagittal fat-suppressed T2-weighted image shows rimlike hyperintense signal similar to fluid at the fragment-bone interface (*arrow*), which suggests instability. (*C*) Twenty-one months later, the patient presents with limitation of elbow extension. A fat-suppressed T2-weighted image now shows a displaced fragment (*arrow*) in the posterior aspect of the elbow joint.

criterion was not sensitive when used alone. They also identified correctly the 3 arthroscopically proven stable lesions in their study population using these criteria, although specificity was not commented on. In contrast, a study by Iwasaki and colleagues[40] performed in overhead athletes also with a mean age of 14 years (but 5 patients between 16 and 20 years of age and 1 patient >20 years of age) found that De Smet and colleagues'[17,18] original criteria had only an 89% sensitivity and 44% specificity for the prediction of fragment instability. MRI performed poorly in the determination of lesion stability compared with surgery as the gold standard, although their study had recognized limitations. These limitations included a small number of patients with preoperative MRI examinations indicating stability and a selection bias in that only patients with surgical correlation were used for the study, thus selecting for a group of patients that had either a more advanced stage of OCD or long-standing symptoms not responsive to conservative treatment.[40]

In addition, clinicians should not confuse an OCD lesion of the capitellum, which typically is in the anterolateral aspect of the capitellum, with the normal anatomic variant referred to as a pseudodefect, which is located more posteriorly between the smooth articular surface of the posterior-inferior capitellum and the adjacent lateral epicondyle (**Fig. 23**).[38]

ANKLE

At the ankle, the broader term osteochondral lesion (OCL) is often used instead of OCD because of the recognition that many of these lesions are the direct result of trauma. The term OCD is reserved for a distinct subset of OCLs that may be associated with a genetic, endocrine, or metabolic abnormality and does not necessarily require a history of antecedent trauma.[41,42] Similar to the elbow, a classification system developed by Berndt and Harty[43] in 1959 based on radiography was used originally to help stage patients with OCLs of the talus. Stage 1 lesions were characterized by focal subchondral trabecular compression; stage 2 by a partially detached fragment; stage 3 by a completely detached, in situ fragment; and stage 4 by a detached

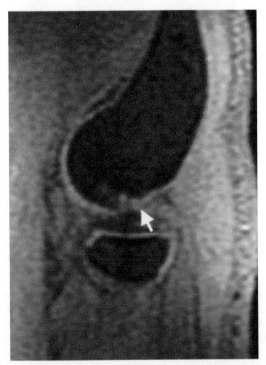

Fig. 23. Pseudodefect of the capitellum. Sagittal 3D fat-suppressed T1-weighted gradient echo image shows irregularity (*arrow*) at the junction of the posteroinferior capitellum and adjacent lateral epicondyle, the characteristic site and appearance of a pseudodefect.

and displaced fragment. Similar to other radiographically based classification systems, its strength lies in its simplicity; however, like other radiographically based systems, subsequent studies have shown that it is not very sensitive, with up to 50% of OCLs not detected on conventional radiographs.[42] Numerous staging systems were subsequently proposed between 1986 and 2003, which include a modification to Berndt and Harty's[43] original system, as well as systems based on arthroscopy, computed tomography (CT), and most commonly MRI.[19,44–48]

OCLs of the talus were classically described to occur in the anterolateral and posteromedial talar dome; however, recent studies that used MRI have shown that most lesions are located medially and centrally, followed by a lateral and central location.[49,50] Although most commonly seen in the talar dome, OCLs may involve many other sites about the ankle, which include the talar head, tibial plafond, cuboid, navicular, subtalar joint, and various metatarsal heads.[41]

On CT, subchondral cystlike foci, as well as detachment, fragmentation, and displacement of bone fragments, are features that suggest instability (**Fig. 24**). Despite the usefulness of CT to provide additional characterization of an OCL, MRI is the preferred modality because of its ability to visualize abnormality in adjacent bone marrow and overlying cartilage, which results in improved sensitivity for early stage OCLs.[41] MRI is often ordered in the clinical setting of a conservatively treated ankle sprain with prolonged pain refractory to treatment and normal radiographs to assess for a radiographically occult OCL.[41]

Early OCLs may manifest simply as a focal area of bone marrow edema pattern, sometimes flame shaped, on T2-weighted images at one side of a joint.[41] However, MRI may overestimate the severity of injury within the bone, and a bone marrow edema pattern does not necessarily indicate acuity of injury. Bone marrow edema pattern can be seen acutely in the setting of a bone bruise as well as chronically in the setting of reactive marrow changes related to long-standing instability or osteoarthritis, among other causes.[42]

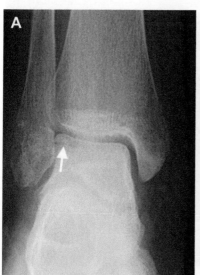 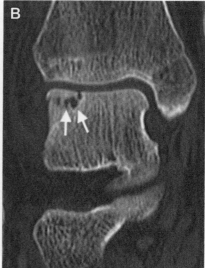

Fig. 24. Unstable talar osteochondral lesion. (*A*) AP radiograph shows an osteochondral lesion (*arrow*) of the lateral talar dome. (*B*) Coronal CT reformation better reveals cystlike foci (*arrows*) at the base of the OCL in this surgically proven unstable lesion.

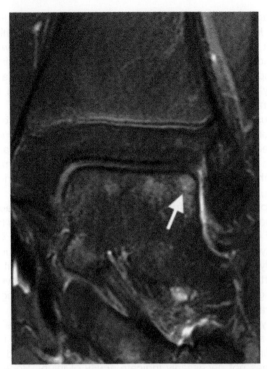

Fig. 25. Stable talar osteochondral lesion. Coronal fat-suppressed T2-weighted image shows subchondral marrow edema pattern (*arrow*) of the lateral talar dome, indicating a low-grade OCL.

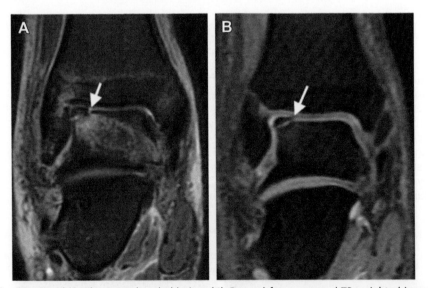

Fig. 26. Unstable talar osteochondral lesion. (*A*) Coronal fat-suppressed T2-weighted image shows a fissure containing fluid signal intensity (*arrow*) at the medial margin of the OCL, with discontinuity of the subchondral bone. (*B*) The same fissure (*arrow*) but with disruption of the hyperintense signal articular cartilage on a fat-suppressed 3D T1-weighted GRE sequence.

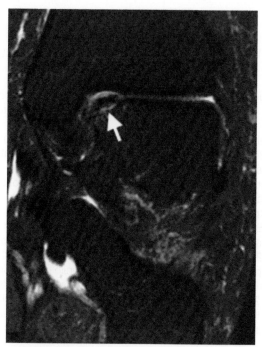

Fig. 27. Unstable osteochondral lesion. Coronal fat-suppressed T2-weighted image shows a hyperintense T2 signal rim (*arrow*) similar to fluid signal intensity at the fragment-bone interface.

Accurate description and assessment of OCL stability is a useful goal for MRI evaluation. De Smet and colleagues[17] original criteria for lesions of the knee are applicable to lesions of the ankle, and may be used to provide imaging support for the diagnosis of instability. Similar to the original Berndt and Harty[43] classification system, bone marrow edema pattern indicates subchondral compression or bone bruise, but without other abnormality it suggests a mild or early stage OCL (**Fig. 25**). In a similar way, articular cartilage damage either characterized by hyperintense signal on T2-weighted images or surface fibrillation typically is present in an earlier stage OCL, whereas deeper fissures that extend to bone, cystlike foci, or a hyperintense rim on T2-weighted images that indicate a loose, but nondisplaced fragment suggest a later stage OCL (**Figs. 26** and **27**). Other features that may suggest instability include extensive bone marrow edema pattern out of proportion to any recent trauma, or interval collapse of the articular surface since the initial injury.[41]

SUMMARY

Various imaging modalities can be used as important adjuncts to a physical examination and surgical therapy in the treatment of patients with OCD. Both radiographs and MRI can be used to aid in diagnosis, to define a treatment plan, to monitor progress, to assess surgical intervention, and to identify postoperative complications. In addition to well-established imaging techniques, newer MRI sequences may hold promise for objective evaluation of tissue composition and integrity.

REFERENCES

1. Clanton TO, DeLee JC. Osteochondritis dissecans. History, pathophysiology and current treatment concepts. Clin Orthop Relat Res 1982;(167):50–64.
2. Glancy GL. Juvenile osteochondritis dissecans. Am J Knee Surg 1999;12(2): 120–4.
3. Hefti F, Beguiristain J, Krauspe R, et al. Osteochondritis dissecans: a multicenter study of the European Pediatric Orthopedic Society. J Pediatr Orthop B 1999; 8(4):231–45.
4. Pill SG, Ganley TJ, Milam RA, et al. Role of magnetic resonance imaging and clinical criteria in predicting successful nonoperative treatment of osteochondritis dissecans in children. J Pediatr Orthop 2003;23(1):102–8.
5. Wall EJ, Vourazeris J, Myer GD, et al. The healing potential of stable juvenile osteochondritis dissecans knee lesions. J Bone Joint Surg Am 2008;90(12): 2655–64. http://dx.doi.org/10.2106/JBJS.G.01103.
6. Kijowski R, Blankenbaker DG, Shinki K, et al. Juvenile versus adult osteochondritis dissecans of the knee: appropriate MR imaging criteria for instability. Radiology 2008;248(2):571–8. http://dx.doi.org/10.1148/radiol.2482071234.
7. Laor T, Zbojniewicz AM, Eismann EA, et al. Juvenile osteochondritis dissecans: is it a growth disturbance of the secondary physis of the epiphysis? AJR Am J Roentgenol 2012;199(5):1121–8. http://dx.doi.org/10.2214/AJR.11.8085.
8. Chambers HG, Shea KG, Carey JL. AAOS clinical practice guideline: diagnosis and treatment of osteochondritis dissecans. J Am Acad Orthop Surg 2011; 19(5):307–9.
9. Moktassi A, Popkin CA, White LM, et al. Imaging of osteochondritis dissecans. Orthop Clin North Am 2012;43(2):201–11. http://dx.doi.org/10.1016/j.ocl.2012. 01.001, v–vi.
10. Sontag LW, Pyle SI. Variations in the calcification pattern in epiphyses. AJR Am J Roentgenol 1941;45:50–4.
11. Caffey J, Madell SH, Royer C, et al. Ossification of the distal femoral epiphysis. J Bone Joint Surg Am 1958;40-A(3):647–54 passim.
12. Nawata K, Teshima R, Morio Y, et al. Anomalies of ossification in the posterolateral femoral condyle: assessment by MRI. Pediatr Radiol 1999;29(10):781–4.
13. Gebarski K, Hernandez RJ. Stage-I osteochondritis dissecans versus normal variants of ossification in the knee in children. Pediatr Radiol 2005;35(9): 880–6. http://dx.doi.org/10.1007/s00247-005-1507-6.
14. Jans LB, Jaremko JL, Ditchfield M, et al. MRI differentiates femoral condylar ossification evolution from osteochondritis dissecans. A new sign. Eur Radiol 2011;21(6):1170–9. http://dx.doi.org/10.1007/s00330-011-2058-x.
15. Jans LB, Jaremko JL, Ditchfield M, et al. Evolution of femoral condylar ossification at MR imaging: frequency and patient age distribution. Radiology 2011; 258(3):880–8. http://dx.doi.org/10.1148/radiol.10101103.
16. Jans L, Jaremko J, Ditchfield M, et al. Ossification variants of the femoral condyles are not associated with osteochondritis dissecans. Eur J Radiol 2012; 81(11):3384–9. http://dx.doi.org/10.1016/j.ejrad.2012.01.009.
17. De Smet AA, Fisher DR, Graf BK, et al. Osteochondritis dissecans of the knee: value of MR imaging in determining lesion stability and the presence of articular cartilage defects. AJR Am J Roentgenol 1990;155(3):549–53. http://dx.doi.org/ 10.2214/ajr.155.3.2117355.
18. De Smet AA, Ilahi OA, Graf BK. Reassessment of the MR criteria for stability of osteochondritis dissecans in the knee and ankle. Skeletal Radiol 1996;25(2):159–63.

19. Dipaola JD, Nelson DW, Colville MR. Characterizing osteochondral lesions by magnetic resonance imaging. Arthroscopy 1991;7(1):101–4.
20. Heywood CS, Benke MT, Brindle K, et al. Correlation of magnetic resonance imaging to arthroscopic findings of stability in juvenile osteochondritis dissecans. Arthroscopy 2011;27(2):194–9. http://dx.doi.org/10.1016/j.arthro.2010.07.009.
21. Mesgarzadeh M, Sapega AA, Bonakdarpour A, et al. Osteochondritis dissecans: analysis of mechanical stability with radiography, scintigraphy, and MR imaging. Radiology 1987;165(3):775–80. http://dx.doi.org/10.1148/radiology.165.3.3685359.
22. Nelson DW, DiPaola J, Colville M, et al. Osteochondritis dissecans of the talus and knee: prospective comparison of MR and arthroscopic classifications. J Comput Assist Tomogr 1990;14(5):804–8.
23. O'Connor MA, Palaniappan M, Khan N, et al. Osteochondritis dissecans of the knee in children. A comparison of MRI and arthroscopic findings. J Bone Joint Surg Br 2002;84(2):258–62.
24. Samora WP, Chevillet J, Adler B, et al. Juvenile osteochondritis dissecans of the knee: predictors of lesion stability. J Pediatr Orthop 2012;32(1):1–4. http://dx.doi.org/10.1097/BPO.0b013e31823d8312.
25. Yoshida S, Ikata T, Takai H, et al. Osteochondritis dissecans of the femoral condyle in the growth stage. Clin Orthop Relat Res 1998;(346):162–70.
26. Krause M, Hapfelmeier A, Moller M, et al. Healing predictors of stable juvenile osteochondritis dissecans knee lesions after 6 and 12 months of nonoperative treatment. Am J Sports Med 2013;41(10):2384–91. http://dx.doi.org/10.1177/0363546513496049.
27. Parikh SN, Allen M, Wall EJ, et al. The reliability to determine "healing" in osteochondritis dissecans from radiographic assessment. J Pediatr Orthop 2012;32(6):e35–9. http://dx.doi.org/10.1097/BPO.0b013e31825fa80f.
28. Choi YS, Potter HG, Chun TJ. MR imaging of cartilage repair in the knee and ankle. Radiographics 2008;28(4):1043–59. http://dx.doi.org/10.1148/rg.284075111.
29. Behery O, Siston RA, Harris JD, et al. Treatment of cartilage defects of the knee: expanding on the existing algorithm. Clin J Sport Med 2013. http://dx.doi.org/10.1097/JSM.0000000000000004.
30. Hayter C, Potter H. Magnetic resonance imaging of cartilage repair techniques. J Knee Surg 2011;24(4):225–40.
31. Bartlett W, Gooding CR, Carrington RWJ, et al. Autologous chondrocyte implantation at the knee using a bilayer collagen membrane with bone graft. J Bone Joint Surg (Br) 2005;87-B:330–2.
32. Sirlin CB, Boutin RD, Brossmann J, et al. Polydioxanone biodegradable pins in the knee: MR imaging. AJR Am J Roentgenol 2001;176(1):83–90. http://dx.doi.org/10.2214/ajr.176.1.1760083.
33. Crema MD, Roemer FW, Marra MD, et al. Articular cartilage in the knee: current MR imaging techniques and applications in clinical practice and research. Radiographics 2011;31(1):37–61. http://dx.doi.org/10.1148/rg.311105084.
34. Potter HG, Black BR, Chong le R. New techniques in articular cartilage imaging. Clin Sports Med 2009;28(1):77–94. http://dx.doi.org/10.1016/j.csm.2008.08.004.
35. Baker CL 3rd, Romeo AA, Baker CL Jr. Osteochondritis dissecans of the capitellum. Am J Sports Med 2010;38(9):1917–28. http://dx.doi.org/10.1177/0363546509354969.
36. Janarv PM, Hesser U, Hirsch G. Osteochondral lesions in the radiocapitellar joint in the skeletally immature: radiographic, MRI, and arthroscopic findings in 13 consecutive cases. J Pediatr Orthop 1997;17(3):311–4.

37. Kijowski R, De Smet AA. Radiography of the elbow for evaluation of patients with osteochondritis dissecans of the capitellum. Skeletal Radiol 2005;34(5):266–71. http://dx.doi.org/10.1007/s00256-005-0899-6.

38. Kijowski R, De Smet AA. MRI findings of osteochondritis dissecans of the capitellum with surgical correlation. AJR Am J Roentgenol 2005;185(6):1453–9. http://dx.doi.org/10.2214/AJR.04.1570.

39. Jans LB, Ditchfield M, Anna G, et al. MR imaging findings and MR criteria for instability in osteochondritis dissecans of the elbow in children. Eur J Radiol 2012;81(6):1306–10. http://dx.doi.org/10.1016/j.ejrad.2011.01.007.

40. Iwasaki N, Kamishima T, Kato H, et al. A retrospective evaluation of magnetic resonance imaging effectiveness on capitellar osteochondritis dissecans among overhead athletes. Am J Sports Med 2012;40(3):624–30. http://dx.doi.org/10.1177/0363546511429258.

41. Naran KN, Zoga AC. Osteochondral lesions about the ankle. Radiol Clin North Am 2008;46(6):995–1002. http://dx.doi.org/10.1016/j.rcl.2008.10.001, v.

42. O'Loughlin PF, Heyworth BE, Kennedy JG. Current concepts in the diagnosis and treatment of osteochondral lesions of the ankle. Am J Sports Med 2010; 38(2):392–404. http://dx.doi.org/10.1177/0363546509336336.

43. Berndt A, Harty M. Transchondral fractures (osteochondritis dissecans) of the talus. J Bone Joint Surg Am 1959;41-A:988–1020.

44. Ferkel RD, Zanotti RM, Komenda GA, et al. Arthroscopic treatment of chronic osteochondral lesions of the talus: long-term results. Am J Sports Med 2008; 36(9):1750–62. http://dx.doi.org/10.1177/0363546508316773.

45. Hepple S, Winson IG, Glew D. Osteochondral lesions of the talus: a revised classification. Foot Ankle Int 1999;20(12):789–93.

46. Mintz DN, Tashjian GS, Connell DA, et al. Osteochondral lesions of the talus: a new magnetic resonance grading system with arthroscopic correlation. Arthroscopy 2003;19(4):353–9. http://dx.doi.org/10.1053/jars.2003.50041.

47. Pritsch M, Horoshovski H, Farine I. Arthroscopic treatment of osteochondral lesions of the talus. J Bone Joint Surg Am 1986;68(6):862–5.

48. Taranow WS, Bisignani GA, Towers JD, et al. Retrograde drilling of osteochondral lesions of the medial talar dome. Foot Ankle Int 1999;20(8):474–80.

49. Elias I, Zoga AC, Morrison WB, et al. Osteochondral lesions of the talus: localization and morphologic data from 424 patients using a novel anatomical grid scheme. Foot Ankle Int 2007;28(2):154–61. http://dx.doi.org/10.3113/FAI.2007.0154.

50. Hembree WC, Wittstein JR, Vinson EN, et al. Magnetic resonance imaging features of osteochondral lesions of the talus. Foot Ankle Int 2012;33(7):591–7. http://dx.doi.org/10.3113/FAI.2012.0001.

Osteochondritis Dissecans of the Elbow

Carl W. Nissen, MD

KEYWORDS

- Osteochondritis dissecans • Elbow • Adolescent sports

KEY POINTS

- Osteochondritis dissecans (OCD) of the elbow, usually of the capitellum, is the second most common location seen in young, athletic individuals.
- Some sports seem to increase the risk of elbow OCD: overhead sports, such as baseball, and upper extremity weight-bearing sports, such as gymnastics.
- Elbow OCD is often diagnosed after the chondral surface has been significantly compromised and this lessens the chance to preserve them.

INTRODUCTION

Osteochondritis dissecans (OCD) is a musculoskeletal problem occurring primarily in the maturing skeleton. Many early descriptions of the problem came from surgeons who opened the knee joint looking for the cause of catching and locking symptoms. In these first cases, large, loose OCD fragments were found and removed, making the patients significantly better in the short run, although often not in the long-term.[1] To describe the pathology, Konig in 1887 coined the phrase "osteochondritis dissecans." Many authors disagreed with his description and attempts to change the name occurred for years.[2] The difference between the juvenile and adult forms of the disease also led to significant differing opinions about the problem and its best treatment.[3] Improvements in imaging and especially the emergence of magnetic resonance imaging (MRI) sequences in the diagnosis and care of OCD have led to an improved understanding and ability to treat the problem. The most recent definition of human OCD lesions, proposed by the Research in Osteochondritis of the Knee study group, highlights that these are (1) focal; (2) idiopathic; (3) involve subchondral bone; and (4) risk instability and disruption of articular cartilage with potential long-term consequences, such as premature osteoarthritis.[4] There are still many unanswered questions, however, with regards to the cause and the best treatment options for OCD when diagnosed.

Elite Sports Medicine, 399 Farmington Ave, Farmington, CT 06032, USA; Department of Orthopaedics, University of Connecticut, 263 Farmington Avenue, Farmington, CT 06030, USA
E-mail address: cnissen@connecticutchildrens.org

Clin Sports Med 33 (2014) 251–265
http://dx.doi.org/10.1016/j.csm.2013.11.002   sportsmed.theclinics.com

The original description of OCD and the most common location for it is within the maturing knee along the lateral border of the medial femoral condyle with an overall incidence of these lesions in the knee reported to be between 18 (females) and 29 (males) per 100,000.[5] Linden and colleagues[5] noted the incidence to seemingly be increasing and others have noted a simultaneously decreasing age at presentation.[3,6] OCD is also increasingly diagnosed in other joints, such as ankle, hip, elbow, and shoulder. The elbow in particular, where OCD is most commonly seen in the capitellum, is increasing in incidence at the most rapid rate.[7]

The increased incidence and therefore interest in capitellar OCD has paralleled the increased competitive, year-round involvement of young athletes in upper extremity–dominant sports. The use of high-resolution MRI allows earlier diagnosis of the problem and the ability to differentiate OCD from osteonecrosis; osteochondrosis; hereditary epiphyseal dysplasia; little leaguer's elbow; and most importantly, Panner disease, an articular osteochondrosis of the capitellum,[8] with which it is often confused.[9–11] Compared with Panner disease, where patients are often prepubescent with full resolution of the problem and a good clinical outcome, the outcome for capitellar OCD is not always good with the prognosis and outcome dependent on the patient age, location, and severity at the time of diagnosis.[12–14] Sports placing repetitive weight-bearing stress on the elbow, such as gymnastics, or repetitive compression forces seen in overhead athletes, such as baseball players or javelin throwers, lead to articular cartilage changes and stress reaction to the subchondral bone. This starts a cascade of events that can lead to or propagate an OCD lesion. Although many of these lesions can heal, a delay in diagnosis with continued stressing of the lesion interferes with this healing and can lead to long-term consequences and worsening of elbow function.

ETIOLOGY AND DISEASE PROGRESSION

After the inflammatory cause of OCD was discounted authors shifted their attention to other possibilities.[15,16] Some evidence does exist for there to be a genetic predisposition in OCD within the knee but this cause in the elbow has not been shown.[17] OCD within the elbow seems to be related to repetitive microtrauma, which leads to a perpetuation of an established lesion or perhaps its creation. This is supported by the correlation seen between sports where the upper extremity is weight bearing (gymnastics and wrestling) or where repetitive joint loading (baseball and javelin) occurs. Reviewing the correlation between OCD lesions and these sports[18] seems to confirm repetitive trauma as a major cause of elbow OCD.[9]

After the pathologic process has started most authors acknowledge that the healing potential of OCD, especially when present in the capitellum, is limited because of the tenuous blood supply of the capitellum. This is a relative deviation away from knee OCD where the blood supply of the distal femur is excellent. In the case of the knee the plasticity and health of the young, growing bone allows it to heal with no long-term morbidity when put into the right environment at an early stage of the disease. Conversely, if the elbow is subjected to ongoing stress the tenuous blood supply of the capitellum does not allow the bone to heal and an unfortunate cascade of events occurs making it similar to the process of avascular necrosis seen in femoral and humeral heads.[19] In these situations the subchondral bone softens leading to a loss of a solid foundation for the overlying articular cartilage. The cartilage fissures, exposing the bone to synovial fluid, which leads to further bone injury and further deterioration as the synovial and inflammatory fluid tracks beneath the subchondral bone. This lessens the chance for bony healing to occur and increases the chance that the bone will fragment forming progeny bone within the capitellar OCD crater. As the disease progresses the nonhealing progeny bone becomes a loose fragment ultimately leading to the locking of the elbow as was seen in the knee when the disease was first described.

At this point no universally accepted classification systems exist for OCD. As research into OCD continues classification systems based on physical examination, radiograph, and MRI findings, and then ultimately arthroscopic findings will be established allowing many of the current ideas regarding disease progression and steps in OCD management to be studied and established.

PRESENTATION AND DIAGNOSIS

Young athletes with capitellar OCD often have diffuse, nonspecific complaints that center on activity with mild, inflammatory-like symptoms after exercise. Rest and anti-inflammatory treatment is effective for their symptoms early in the disease process, which is perhaps the reason that there is often a delay in presentation and diagnosis. It is uncommon that a patient with elbow OCD comes in without some report of a prodrome. Resting or modifying activity for a week or two often resolves an athlete's pain completely leading them to believe they had a minor strain that has healed. Year-round athletes often try to work through the pain, managing their pain symptomatically, and they often have several episodes of pain throughout the year waiting to seek medical advice until they feel catching and sharp pain during their activity. Multisport athletes often treat their pain symptomatically until the offending sport season ends. They then participate in less elbow stressful sports, but once the offending sport season returns, their pain also returns. It is often not until this point-in-time that their performance starts to suffer and they may have additional symptoms, such as an effusion and a loss of terminal extension that can also interfere with everyday activities. Once the lesion is advanced where a loose fragment exists, a noticeable click or even locking may be present and is an ominous sign in these athletes. Additionally, the author has found that the existence of pain while performing their sport, such as while the ball is in a pitcher's hand before ball release, is predictably a sign that the OCD lesion has become mechanical in nature and the likelihood of healing, even with appropriate rest and nonoperative care, is slight.

The physical examination in OCD cases focuses on the patient's range-of-motion including supination and pronation, examination for any effusion, a ligamentous examination focusing on ulnar collateral insufficiency and radiocapitellar rotatory instability, and palpable tenderness about the elbow especially in the posterolateral corner.

Because many athletes appear in the office for their examination after or during a period of rest the chance of obvious pathology on examination is reduced. In these instances we often attempt to exercise the patients to improve the diagnostic ability of the examination. As an example, for baseball players we ask them to throw outside or in the gym to stir up their discomfort. We do so only after we confirm that no large loose fragment exists in the joint and that at least near full range-of-motion and good strength exists.

Standard elbow radiographs should be taken including oblique views of the elbow (radial head views) to look for OCD of the capitellum. The taking of the anteroposterior view at 90 degrees to the shaft of the humerus and angling the x-ray beam 30 degrees cephalad allows more of the capitellar surface to be visualized, similar to the Rosenberg views of the knee. We also take an axillary view of the elbow, similar to a Merchant view of the knee (**Figs. 1–4**). Although the boney architecture is usually

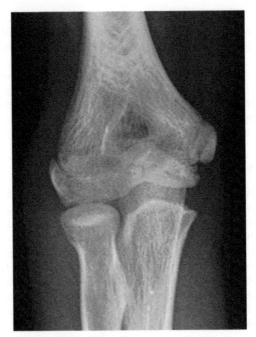

Fig. 1. Anteroposterior radiograph of the elbow.

determined by radiograph, occasionally a CT scan is helpful to better define the subchondral bone condition (**Fig. 5**).

The imaging modality of choice for OCD of the elbow is an MRI. The MRI allows an evaluation of the articular cartilage and underlying bone. The prognostic ability of an MRI in these cases has not been worked out yet but the ability to see many of the finer details of the lesion is possible. It is particularly helpful in determining the acuity of the process by noting the presence or absence of bony edema. Additional information, such as the separation of the progeny bone from the native bone, the loss of articular cartilage continuity, the tracking of synovial or inflammatory fluid between the progeny and native bone, and especially the viability of the progeny bone, are all extremely helpful in treatment planning. High-field MRI with cartilage sequences is very helpful

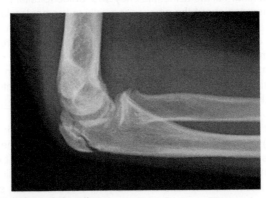

Fig. 2. Lateral radiograph of the elbow.

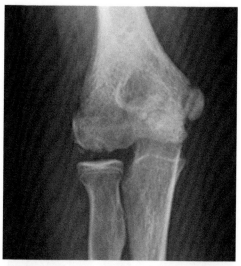

Fig. 3. Oblique radiograph of the elbow. Radiocapitellar joint visualized.

in the evaluation (**Figs. 6** and **7**). The increasing availability of 3-T magnets and the clarity of articular cartilage on these scans will likely help in this portion of the evaluation; however, their use is not clearly defined. Most of our radiology colleagues believe that special sequences performed with a 1.5-T magnet are perhaps more functional at this time. Although not a part of our regular MRI evaluation, MRI arthrograms can be ordered. The use of intra-articular dye is often helpful in evaluating the ulnar collateral ligament of the elbow and to a lesser extent the presence or absence of loose bodies within the joint. In the case of OCD, however, the dye may reduce the usefulness of the

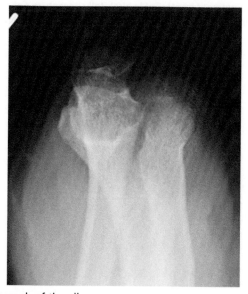

Fig. 4. Axillary radiograph of the elbow.

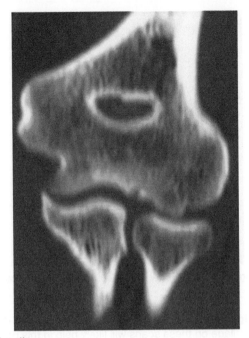

Fig. 5. CT scan of the elbow.

MRI because it decreases the ability to see small chondral fissures and the extent of bony edema.

NONOPERATIVE TREATMENT

Nonoperative treatment when OCD is diagnosed at an early stage can be successful and has been the mainstay of treatment in skeletally immature patients for many years. Successful treatment, either operatively or nonoperatively, requires the reduction or

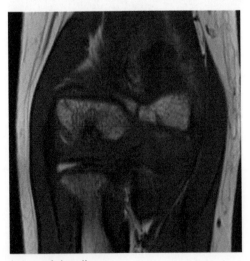

Fig. 6. MRI T2 sagittal view of the elbow.

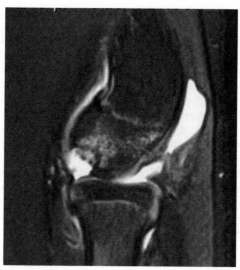

Fig. 7. MRI T2 coronal view of the elbow.

elimination of all stress for a period of at least 6 weeks to allow the subchondral bone to stabilize, heal, and support the overlying cartilage. Deciding when to start a slow and planned progression back into day-to-day functioning and ultimately athletic activities is difficult. Using repeat imaging, although intuitively a good idea, is not established as a viable method to determine return to activities. Furthermore, patients often heal their lesions and return back to full activities despite the lack of full radiographic healing. Many authors suggest that the timeline may be as long as 6 months to allow complete healing.[13] Unfortunately, the ability to prognosticate when conservative treatment will be successful is not well established and the decision to initiate nonoperative management in capitellar OCD focuses on the extent of disease, the time from onset of symptoms, and the patient's expectations and desires. As in the treatment of knee OCD, results of nonoperative treatment are better in younger, prepubescent athletes with wide-open physes.[20] We also believe that if the radiographs or the MRI do not show separation of the fragment with fluid between the native and progeny bone, a period of rest has a decent chance to result in a full functional recovery in at least half of the cases. However, once an athlete complains of clicking or locking regardless of the timeliness of diagnosis and their age, the likelihood that conservative management will be successful decreases.

When rest is difficult to accomplish, bracing, use of a sling, or even a period of casting is used. We are very careful with this treatment arm of the algorithm, however, because the elbow losses functional range-of-motion faster than most joints in the body when it is immobilized. Return to activities is appropriate only after there is complete resolution of symptoms and the athlete has regained full range-of-motion and strength not only about the elbow but also of the shoulder girdle.[1]

OPERATIVE TREATMENT

When nonoperative treatment is unsuccessful or the OCD progeny fragment is loose, operative treatment is appropriate. Although some historical and physical examination findings clearly point to operative management, these are not always present and sometimes the decision to take a patient to the operating room needs to be individualized. Ultimately the goal of treatment once initiated is to preserve functional ability in the long-term and to halt progression of the disease and especially not allow a free chondral or bony fragment to occur. In our experience, capitellar OCD operative treatment is often delayed resulting in the finding of such a loose fragment. We have become more aggressive in this entity using a series of attributes of the lesion to help with the decision to operate, such as presence of clicking or locking; loss of terminal extension; pain during activity; position of the lesion, especially the involvement of the lateral border of the capitellum; depth of the lesion; and timing of the athlete's next season. Ultimately, however, a significant amount of further research is needed to define the point when transitioning to operative management is appropriate.

Surgery can be performed in the prone, lateral, or supine position. Each has advantages for accessibility to the elbow. The prone position does allow the neurovascular structures to fall away relatively from the surgical field, although the position creates a change in spatial arrangement from the anatomic position. Additionally, although anesthesia is certainly possible for individuals in the prone position, most anesthesiologists favor lateral and supine positioning.

Appropriate OCD treatment is determined by future demands of the patient and staging of the lesion that includes preoperative symptoms, appearance on imaging studies, and arthroscopic appearance of the lesion. Many options are available, although few controlled trials exist to help determine the best option.[21]

In cases when the lesion is in an early stage of development, most options center on helping the subchondral bone to heal. When there is no break or fissuring in the articular surface, drilling of the reactive bone has been reported to achieve excellent short-term results.[22–26] The drilling can be done either transarticular or extra-articular depending on the accessibility of the lesion and its extent. The elbow must be allowed to rest after the drilling so that the bone stabilizes before weight-bearing or repetitive activities are instituted. When done early in the disease process, these lesions do very well and a full return to premorbid levels of activity is often achieved. However, longer-term follow-up studies have revealed some concern regarding the continuation of high-level activities and the possibility of developing degenerative joint disease in these cases of drilling.[12,14,27]

When visualization of the lesion demonstrates the OCD to be further along the continuum with the presence of articular cartilage fissures or the OCD progeny bone demonstrates characteristics that it is separating from the native bone an attempt to preserve the fragment is recommended (**Fig. 8**). This can be achieved

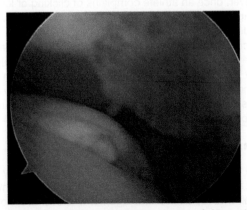

Fig. 8. Arthroscopic view of loose but in situ OCD progeny of the capitellum.

with a myriad of devices including bioabsorbable pins or screws, metal screws, bone dowels, osteochondral plugs, or direct suturing of the fragment.[9,21] This approach, when possible, coupled with appropriate postoperative rest and rehabilitation, can lead to excellent long-term results. Again, however, the criteria on which to make the decision to perform fixation of the lesion have not been determined.[1]

If the fragment is loose, preparation of the bed and often bone grafting is necessary. When the fragment has not become swollen and can still fit snuggly in the crater and has some bone on it, the chances of achieving a good result with fixation exist. Although possible arthroscopically, making an arthrotomy to perform either open bone grafting and repair may be needed in these cases.[7,28,29]

When the fragment is dislodged and unable to be fixed (**Fig. 9**), excision of the fragment and meticulous debridement is performed to remove fibrocartilage to enhance the chance for the lesion to fill in. This does provide good pain relief in the short run and improvement of function when the lesion is contained (**Figs. 10** and **11**).[22,30–32] Postoperative MRIs in these cases do demonstrate the ability for fibrocartilage to fill the defect.[33] However, several authors have shown that long-term results of fragment excision with or without marrow stimulation often lead to recurrent loose bodies, degenerative changes, and capitellar remodeling.[34]

Longer-term follow-up studies should allow a better understanding of when fragment excision and debridement can lead to good results versus the need to perform fixation or transplantation to restore full functional ability and help prevent long-term problems. One subgroup of individuals that seem to have poorer long-term results is those with lesions that extend beyond the shoulder of the capitellum.[35] By losing the lateral support for the radial head during activities it is theorized that increased stress and some level of instability across the joint occurs. Re-establishing the lateral border or column with bony support and an intact cartilage surface may reduce long-term functional problems. Achieving this with osteochondral autograft reconstruction of the capitellum in several early term reports has demonstrated the ability to return patients to a high functional level and often premorbid levels of activity (**Fig. 12**).[29,36–40] Obtaining osteochondral plugs from the patient's knee is often needed to accomplish this, because suitable grafts are not easily obtained within the elbow. The morbidity of obtaining these grafts is not without concern[41,42] and this has led to the suggestion that either that osteochondral allografting procedures should be considered[43] or alternatively osteochondral autografting from a rib.[44]

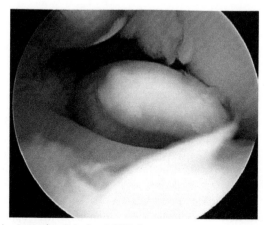

Fig. 9. Arthroscopic view of a dislodged OCD fragment.

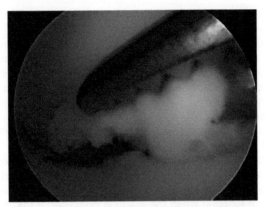

Fig. 10. Grasping of typical loose, disintegrating fragment of capitellar OCD lesion.

Long-term follow-up of these procedures is not yet known.[36,45] The appealing theoretical aspects of these complete-care approaches needs to be compared and contrasted with the long-term outcome and morbidity at the donor site and concerns regarding the use of allograft tissue. Several knee OCD articles have attempted to look at this, although the answer in the case of the knee still is not fully understood.[46]

Some authors have suggested distal humeral osteotomies and although older, these authors have reported excellent results.[47,48] As with other treatment modalities, the morbidity of the treatment needs to be contrasted with the long-term results once known. The rate of return to sports after distal humeral osteotomies in one study was favorable, although recent studies are lacking.[48]

AUTHOR'S SURGICAL PROCEDURE OF CHOICE

Each of our procedures starts with a thorough examination under anesthesia. Although not common in elbow cases, an increased or decreased range-of-motion compared with the office examination is sometimes found and is important with regards to postoperative therapy. Repeat ligamentous examination is also invaluable and a privilege of taking patients to the operating room of which one should take advantage.

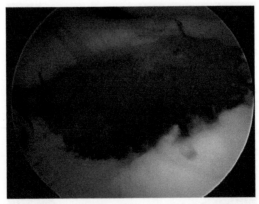

Fig. 11. Arthroscopic view of capitellar OCD lesion base with appropriate early clot formation.

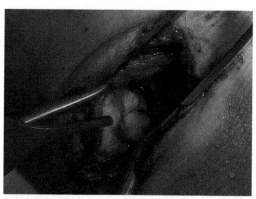

Fig. 12. Capitellar OCD with osteochondral grafts in place.

In our hands the patient is positioned supine with the use of an upper extremity positioner (Spider; Smith and Nephew, Mansfield, MA) (**Fig. 13**). We have found that treatment of all OCD lesions on the capitellum and throughout the elbow is possible using this approach. This includes the treatment of a very anteriorly based OCD of the capitellum.

After the examination under anesthesia, we insufflate the joint with 10 to 15 mL of normal saline through the posterolateral soft spot before establishing the proximal medial portal with a long 2.7-mm arthroscope. In smaller patients and especially when working in the posterior aspect of the elbow, we often switch to a 2.7-mm short arthroscope. A lateral portal is then created under direct vision. It should be noted that this portal is significantly more anterior on the lateral side of the elbow than might intuitively seem appropriate. This portal is established with an exchange rod. This allows us to move between the medial and lateral portals for visualization and treatment with less concern because of the creation of multiple capsular portals accompanied by the potential iatrogenic injuries therewith. After diagnostic and treatment steps are completed anteriorly we use the arm positioner to bring the arm and elbow up over the chest of the patient with the elbow flexed 90 or more degrees. We create a proximal posterolateral portal first at the tip of the olecranon. The camera sheath is passed distally along the surface of the olecranon allowing a clear visualization of the radiocapitellar joint and the capitellar OCD when present. Using a direct soft spot portal to clear scar and soft tissue from the back of the radiocapitellar joint is helpful. This portal is also used to further visualize and examine the lesion. Exchanging the long arthroscope for a shorter scope at this point is helpful. We also have available a full-sized shaver (4 mm) and a thermal ablator because the scar is often difficult to fully debride with the smaller shavers. The arthroscopic procedure includes a careful examination of all surfaces of the elbow because it has been our experience that in long-standing cases of OCD free fragments often become scarred into the synovium and hard to visualize. Because of their potential to effect range-of-motion, these should be recognized and removed with adjacent areas smoothed.

Care of OCD is dictated by the appearance of the lesion arthroscopically with some, but less, input from the preoperative imaging. Lesions with little to no fissuring of the chondral surface are drilled in an extra-articular fashion. This is helped with the use of a small fluoroscope and small targeting device (MicroVector; Smith and Nephew). If there are fissures or the fragment is loose we attempt to preserve fragments even without bone. Fragments without bone if they are substantial enough to hold a suture are sutured into place through a small arthrotomy using 6-0 vicryl sutures. In our

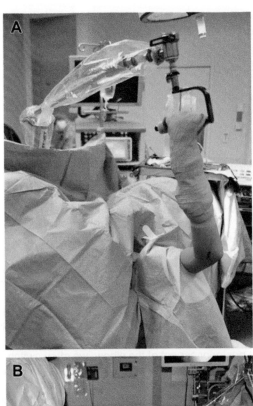

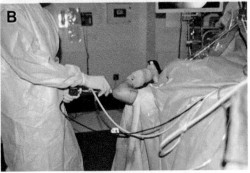

Fig. 13. Elbow arthroscopy set-up as viewed from the head (*A*) and from the foot with elbow in hyperflexion (*B*).

experience, these fragments although void of bone on radiograph or other imaging studies, often when scraped with a scalpel feel rough or gritty indicating the presence of noncalcified or just nonvisible bone. In younger individuals we have noted that this finding is associated with a good potential to achieve healing. After preparing the lesion surface we reattach the fragment similar to suturing a periosteal patch or synthetic membrane in cartilage-preservation procedures.

When the lesion is found to be larger with a definitive piece of bone, fixation is our procedure of choice. We use bioabsorbable screws, although we have no concerns with using metal screws or bone plugs as others have proposed. What we have found, unfortunately, is that regardless of the method of fixation chosen, the results of fixation of these fragments in the capitellum is far inferior to the results of knee OCD fixation procedures.

When the lesion is fragmented or solely chondral in nature and not fixable, we meticulously debride the lesion down to a stable chondral rim and a stable bony bed. If appropriate we also take a chondral biopsy from the tip of the olecranon at this point. We have found as others have that this approach provides not only good short-term relief of symptoms, but additionally, the number of patients treated in this fashion who have returned for recurrent problems or symptoms is few.

When recurrent symptoms do occur we have chosen to treat our younger patients with autografting procedures from the knee. The smaller osteochondral cylinders that currently are available (OATS; Arthrex, Naples, FL) we believe lessen the donor site morbidity and allow us to reconstruct the lesions with structural and mechanically sound implants.

DISCUSSION

The presentation of capitellar OCD is variable and the duration of symptoms before diagnosis is often long. Once diagnosed some basics in the treatment decision process are accepted but few are proved. When a stable capitellar OCD exists, rest is the mainstay of treatment and provided the lesion is not advanced along the continuum of the disease, good results can be anticipated. The length of time for rest must exceed the time needed to eliminate pain for the patient and then an active rehabilitation process can be initiated, although the duration of each of these steps is not established. If the lesion is advanced along the disease continuum and mechanical issues within the elbow exist, delaying surgical intervention is not recommended. In these situations surgery should be directed at stabilizing the fragment if possible or reconstructing it when necessary. As the diagnoses of elbow OCD increase, so too will the collective understanding of these lesions. It is hoped this will lead to better diagnostic, treatment, and ultimately patient outcomes.

REFERENCES

1. Takahara M, Mura N, Sasaki J, et al. Classification, treatment, and outcome of osteochondritis dissecans of the humeral capitellum. J Bone Joint Surg Am 2007; 89(6):1205–14.
2. Barrie HJ. Osteochondritis dissecans 1887-1987. A centennial look at Konig's memorable phrase. J Bone Joint Surg Br 1987;69(5):693–5.
3. Cahill BR. Osteochondritis dissecans of the knee: treatment of juvenile and adult forms. J Am Acad Orthop Surg 1995;3(4):237–47.
4. Edmonds E, Polousky J. A review of knowledge in osteochondritis dissecans: 123 years of minimal evolution from Konig to the ROCK Stuy Group. Clin Orthop Relat Res 2013;471(4):1118–26.
5. Linden B. The incidence of osteochondritis dissecans in the condyles of the femur. Acta Orthop Scand 1976;47(6):664–7.
6. Kocher MS, Tucker R, Ganley T, et al. Management of osteochondritis dissecans of the knee: current concepts review. Am J Sports Med 2006;34:1181.
7. Jones K, Wiesel B, Sankar W, et al. Arthroscopic management of osteochondritis dissecans of the capitellum: mid-term results in adolescent athletes. J Pediatr Orthop 2010;30:8–13.
8. Mitsunga M, Adishian D, Bianco AJ. Osteochondritis of the capitellum. J Trauma 1981;22:53–5.
9. Baker CL, Romeo AA, Baker CL. Osteochondritis dissecans of the capitellum. Am J Sports Med 2010;38(9):1917–28.

10. Bradley JP, Petrie RS. Osteochondritis dissecans of the humeral capitellum. Diagnosis and treatment. Clin Sports Med 2001;20(3):565–90.
11. Shimada K, Yoshida T, Nakata K, et al. Reconstruction with an osteochondral autograft for advanced osteochondritis dissecans of the elbow. Clin Orthop Relat Res 2005;435:140–7.
12. Bauer M, Jonsson K, Josefsson PO, et al. Osteochondritis dissecans of the elbow. A long-term follow-up study. Clin Orthop Relat Res 1992;284:156–60.
13. Takahara M, Ogino T, Fukushima S, et al. Nonoperative treatment of osteochondritis dissecans of the humeral capitellum. Am J Sports Med 1999;27(6):728–32.
14. Takahara M, Ogino T, Sasaki I, et al. Long term outcome of osteochondritis dissecans of the humeral capitellum. Clin Orthop Relat Res 1999;363:108–15.
15. Singer K, Roy S. Osteochondrosis of the humeral capitellum. Am J Sports Med 1984;12:351–60.
16. Schenck RC Jr, Goodnight JM. Osteochondritis dissecans. J Bone Joint Surg Am 1996;78(3):439–56.
17. Petrie PW. Aetiology of osteochondritis dissecans. Failure to establish a familial background. J Bone Joint Surg Br 1977;59(3):366–7.
18. Fleisig GS, Andrews JR, Dillman CJ, et al. Kinetics of baseball pitching with implications about injury mechanisms. Am J Sports Med 1995;23(2):233–9.
19. Haraldsson S. On osteochondrosis deformans juvenilis capituli humeri including investigation of intra-osseous vasculature in distal humerus. Acta Orthop Scand Suppl 1959;38:1–232.
20. Pill S, Ganley T, Milam RA, et al. Role of MRI and clinical criteria in predicting successful nonoperative treatment of osteochondritis dissecans in children. J Pediatr Orthop 2003;23:102–8.
21. Takahara M, Mura N, Sasaki J, et al. Classification, treatment, and outcome os osteochondritis dissecans of the humeral capitellum: surgical technique. J Bone Joint Surg Am 2008;90(Suppl 2 Pt 1):47–62.
22. Byrd JW, Jones KS. Arthroscopic surgery for isolated capitellar osteochondritis dissecans in adolescent baseball players: minimum three-year follow-up. Am J Sports Med 2002;30(4):474–8.
23. Baumgarten TE, Andrews JR, Satterwhite YE. The arthroscopic classification and treatment of osteochondritis dissecans of the capitellum. Am J Sports Med 1998; 26(4):520–3.
24. Tivnon MC, Anzel SH, Waugh TR. Surgical management of osteochondritis dissecans of the capitellum. Am J Sports Med 1976;4(3):121–8.
25. Ruchelsman DE, Hall MP, Youm T. Osteochondritis dissecans of the capitellum: current concepts. J Am Acad Orthop Surg 2010;18(9):557–67.
26. Bojanic I, Ivkovic A, Boric I. Arthroscopy and microfracture technique in the treatment of osteochondritis dissecans of the humeral capitellum: report of three adolescent gymnasts. Knee Surg Sports Traum Arthrosc (Germany) 2006;14:491–6.
27. Mitsunaga MM, Adishian DA, Bianco AJ Jr. Osteochondritis dissecans of the capitellum. J Trauma 1982;22(1):53–5.
28. Harada M, Ogino T, Takahara M, et al. Fragment fixation with a bone graft and dynamic staples for osteochondritis dissecans of the humeral capitellum. J Shoulder Elbow Surg 2002;11(4):368–72.
29. Ahmad CS, Elattrache NS. Treatment of capitellar osteochondritis dissecans. Tech Shoulder Elbow Surg 2006;7(4):169–74.
30. Krijnen MR, Lim L, Willems WJ. Arthroscopic treatment of osteochondritis dissecans of the capitellum: report of 5 female athletes. Arthroscopy 2003;19(2): 210–4.

31. Baumgarten TE. Osteochondritis dissecans of the capitellum. Sports Med Arthrosc Rev 1995;3:219–23.

32. Ruch DS, Cory JW, Poehling GG. The arthroscopic management of osteochondritis dissecans of the adolescent elbow. Arthroscopy 1998;14(8):797–803.

33. Wulf CA, Stone RM, Giveans MR, et al. Magnetic resonance imaging after arthroscopic microfracture of capitellar osteochodritis dissecans. Am J Sports Med 2012;40(11):2549–56.

34. Brownlow H, O'Connor-Read LM, Perko M. Arthroscopic treatment of osteochondritis dissecans of the capitellum. Knee Surg Sports Traumatol Arthrosc 2006;14: 198–202.

35. Shi L, Bae DS, Kocher M, et al. Contained versus uncontained lesions in juvenile elbow osteochondritis dissecans. J Pediatr Orthop 2012;32(3):221–5.

36. Yamamoto Y, Ishibashi Y, Tsuda E, et al. Osteochondral autograft transplantation for osteochondritis dissecans of the elbow in juvenile baseball players: minimum 2-year follow-up. Am J Sports Med 2006;34(5):714–20.

37. Miyamoto W, Yamamoto S, Kii R, et al. Oblique osteochondral plugs transplantation technique for osteochondritis dissecans of the elbow joint. Knee Surg Sports Traumatol Arthrosc 2008;17(2):204–8.

38. Iwasaki N, Kato H, Ishikawa J, et al. Autologous osteochondral mosaicplasty for capitellar osteochondritis dissecans in teenaged patients. Am J Sports Med 2006;34(8):1233–9.

39. Iwasaki N, Kato H, Ishikawa J, et al. Autologous osteochondral mosaicplasty for osteochoindritis dissecans of the elbow in teenage athletes. J Bone Joint Surg Am 2009;91(10):2359–66.

40. Smith MV, Bedi A, Chen N. Surgical treatment for osteochondritis dissecans of the capitellum. Sports Health: A Multidisciplinary Approach 2012;4(5):425–32.

41. Iwasaki N, Kato H, Kamishima T, et al. Donor site evaluation after autologous osteochondral mosaicplasty for cartilaginous lesions of the elbow joint. Am J Sports Med 2007;35(12):2096–100.

42. Reddy S, Pedowitz D, Parekh S, et al. The morbidity associated with osteochondral harvest from asymptomatic knees for the treatment of osteochondral lesions of the talus. Am J Sports Med 2007;35(1):80–5.

43. Nissen C. Osteochondritis dissecans of the elbow. Conn Med 2010;74(8):453–6.

44. Shimada K, Tanaka H, Matsumoto T, et al. Cylindrical costal osteochondral autograft for reconstruction of large defects of the capitellum due to osteochondritis dissecans. J Bone Joint Surg Am 2012;94(11):992–1002.

45. Mihara K, Suzuki K, Makiuchi D, et al. Surgical treatment for osteochondritis dissecans of the humeral capitellum. J Shoulder Elbow Surg 2010;19(1):31–7.

46. Lyon R, Nissen C, Liu X, et al. Can fresh osteochondral allografts restore function in juveniles with osteochondritis dissecans of the knee? Clin Orthop Relat Res 2013;471(4):1166–73.

47. Yoshizu T. Closed wedge osteotomy for osteochondritis dissecans of humeral capitellum (in Japanese). Orthopaedics (Seikeigeka) 1986;37:1232–42.

48. Kiyoshige Y, Takagi M, Yuasa K, et al. Closed-Wedge osteotomy for osteochondritis dissecans of the capitellum. A 7- to 12-year follow-up. Am J Sports Med 2000;28(4):534–7.

Osteochondritis Dissecans of the Talus: Diagnosis and Treatment in Athletes

Paul G. Talusan, MD[a], Matthew D. Milewski, MD[b,c],*,
Jason O. Toy, MD[a], Eric J. Wall, MD[d,e]

KEYWORDS

- Osteochondral lesion • Talus • Osteochondritis dissecans • Osteochondral fracture

KEY POINTS

- Osteochondritis dissecans of the talus is a subset of osteochondral lesions of the talus that also includes osteochondral fractures, avascular necrosis, and degenerative arthritis.
- Immobilization along with activity and weight-bearing modifications remain the first line of treatment of symptomatic stable lesions.
- Retrograde drilling, with or without bone grafting, may be indicated for lesions with intact articular cartilage that have failed conservative treatment.
- Smaller lesions with articular cartilage disruption may do well with fragment excision and marrow stimulation.
- Larger lesions with articular cartilage loss or those that have failed fragment excision and marrow stimulation may be addressed with a variety of salvage procedures including osteochondral autografts, fresh osteochondral allografts, or chondrocyte reimplantation techniques.

INTRODUCTION

Osteochondral lesions of the talus (OLTs) have long perplexed physicians and patients alike. In 1737, Monro[1] first described loose osteochondral fragments within the ankle. Konig's[2] term, osteochondritis dissecans (OCD), was first applied to the ankle by Kappis[3] in 1922. OCD of the talus is a subset of OLT that also includes osteochondral fractures, avascular necrosis, and degenerative arthritis.

Despite decades of treating osteochondral lesions, the causes remain elusive. Various hypotheses exist, including repetitive microtrauma, which may or may not disturb the talar vascularity, as well as nontraumatic causes of vascular disruption

[a] Department of Orthopaedics & Rehabilitation, Yale University School of Medicine, New Haven, CT 06519, USA; [b] Elite Sports Medicine, Connecticut Children's Medical Center, 399 Farmington Avenue, Farmington, CT 06032, USA; [c] Department of Orthopaedics, University of Connecticut, Farmington, CT, USA; [d] Division of Orthopaedic Surgery, Cincinnati Children's Hospital Medical Center, 3333 Burnet Avenue, MLC 2017, Cincinnati, OH, 45229, USA; [e] Department of Surgery, University of Cincinnati School of Medicine, Cincinnati, OH, USA
* Corresponding author.
E-mail address: Mmilewski@connecticutchildrens.org

Clin Sports Med 33 (2014) 267–284
http://dx.doi.org/10.1016/j.csm.2014.01.003
0278-5919/14/$ – see front matter © 2014 Elsevier Inc. All rights reserved.

of the subchondral blood supply. Additionally, there is no consensus regarding the nomenclature. Various terms have been used, such as osteochondral lesion, OCD, osteochondral fracture, and transchondral talus fracture. In an attempt to standardize language for discussing OCD lesions, the Research in Osteochondritis Dissecans of the Knee (ROCK) Group[4] has defined the term OCD as a focal, idiopathic alteration of subchondral bone with risk for instability and disruption of adjacent articular cartilage that may result in premature osteoarthritis.[5] Advances in the diagnosis and management, due in large part to improved imaging modalities, have improved the care and management of these lesions as well as worked to lessen the confusion that exists in regard to them.

INCIDENCE

The exact incidence is unknown; however, a retrospective study among active military personnel estimated an incidence of 27 OLTs per 100,000 person years between 1998 and 2008.[6] Chondral injury may occur in up to 50% of ankle instability episodes.[7–10] Chondral injury may occur in up to 73% of ankle fractures. Fractures of talar body represent approximately 1% of all fractures in some incidence studies.[11,12]

ANATOMY AND PATHOPHYSIOLOGY

Elias and colleagues[13] mapped the talar dome into nine zones (**Fig. 1**) and found that most osteochondral lesions occurred in zone 4 and zone 6, and medial lesions tended to be deeper and occupy a larger surface area. Of note, this study did not distinguish

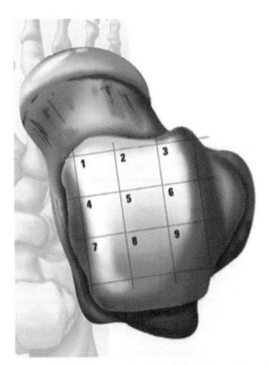

Fig. 1. Anatomic nine-zone grid scheme on the articular surface of the distal tibial plafond. Diagram shows the nine equal surface area zones, with zones 1, 4, and 7 positioned on the medial tibial plafond and zones 1, 2, and 3 positioned anteriorly.

between osteochondral lesions or OCDs. Hembree and colleagues[14] performed a similar study in 77 subjects and found that 54.5% of lesions were centromedial and 31.2% were centrolateral.

Hypotheses regarding the pathophysiology of osteochondral lesions include acute trauma, repeated microtrauma,[15] concomitant ankle instability,[16] vascular insufficiency,[17,18] and genetic predisposition.[17,19–21] Some investigators have divided potential causes into primary and secondary causes.[22,23] An underlying chronic disease of the subchondral bone, possibly due to vascular insufficiency, has been reported by some investigators to be a potential primary cause.[24–26] Secondary causes include trauma, such as ankle fractures or instability, or other external causes.[24–26]

Evidence supporting the hypothesis of vascular insufficiency is lacking. To the authors' knowledge, there are no studies investigating a watershed area of vascularity in the talar dome. A histologic study of osteochondral surgical specimens harvested intraoperatively did not demonstrate areas of subchondral bone necrosis.[27]

DIGiovanni and colleagues[26] examined injuries associated with chronic lateral ankle instability and found that 14 of 60 subjects who underwent an operation for chronic lateral ankle instability had an osteochondral lesion of the talar dome. The investigators did not disclose the location of the lesions; however, 12 of the 14 lesions were chondral flaps requiring debridement and two lesions required debridement and drilling.

Location of the talar lesion may also give us clues to the cause. Most investigators have found a fairly even distribution between medial and lateral talar dome lesions.[7,28] Lateral lesions seem to be associated with trauma nearly 100% of the time, whereas medial lesions are associated with trauma between 64% and 82% of the time.[8,29,30] Medial lesions are usually deep, cup shaped, and associated with subchondral cystic changes. This finding may be related to the increased severity of these lesions and resulting disruption of the subchondral bone plate.[7,31,32]

Although trauma is generally thought to contribute to a large percentage of these lesions, different traumatic mechanisms are described for different lesion locations. Dorsiflexion and inversion with compression is thought to contribute to anterolateral talar dome lesions.[7] Plantar flexion and inversion, with or without external rotation, has been attributed to formation of medial talar dome lesions.[7,33]

HISTORY AND PHYSICAL EXAMINATION

The diagnosis of osteochondral lesions may be elusive during the early stages of patient complaints and can result in a delayed diagnosis.[33] Patients may report an initial trauma with an inversion injury that resolves after a few weeks but may evolve into chronic pain, stiffness, instability, or locking.[15,33] Ironically, a history of antecedent trauma is not necessary.[33] Patients typically report exacerbation of symptoms with weight bearing and activity.[34] Loomer and colleagues[35] reported on 92 adult subjects with OLTs. Eighty nine percent reported a previous ankle injury, 94% had pain with activity, and more than two-thirds reported ankle swelling. Few subjects reported catching, locking, and instability. In skeletally immature subjects, pain is the predominant presentation with few other clinical indicators. In a study of skeletally immature subjects with OCD lesions of the talus, Perumal and colleagues[36] found that 97% of subjects reported pain as a predominant symptom. None of the subjects reported locking or instability, whereas 19% presented with decreased ankle range of motion. Similarly, in a retrospective review of 24 children treated for OCD lesions, 92% presented with pain, followed by swelling in 46%, locking in 8%, and inability to bear weight in 4%.[37] Most patients who present with OCD of the talus present with anterior joint line tenderness. They rarely show an ankle effusion on examination. The talar dome should be palpated with the ankle in both dorsiflexion and plantar flexion. Ankle stability can be assessed with an anterior and posterior drawer test as well as inversion and eversion testing. Ankle plantar flexion and dorsiflexion motion should be compared with the uninvolved ankle in both passive and active modes. In addition, subtalar motion of both ankles must be assessed to determine whether a subtalar coalition exists. This examination is enhanced and made more specific by grasping the heel with the ankle held in dorsiflexion. The medial and lateral ankle ligaments should be checked for tenderness to identify an ankle sprain. The patient's ankle is usually diffusely tender and patients rarely localize their tenderness to the exact location of the OCD on their talus, although localizing the pain in addition to having an effusion has been reported.[15] Loomer and colleagues[35] reported that 15% of subjects had detectable swelling and 19% had an anterior drawer sign. Fifty percent had a loss of ankle dorsiflexion and 20% had detectable loss of subtalar motion.

Because talar OCDs are relatively uncommon, the clinician should consider other more common causes of ankle pain, such as a syndesmotic injury, impingement syndromes, arthritis, occult fracture, lateral ankle instability, tarsal coalition, and subtalar pathologic condition, in the differential diagnosis.[38]

IMAGING AND CLASSIFICATION

The initial imaging modality in patients with ankle pain is a weight-bearing anteroposterior (AP), lateral, and mortise set of radiographs. Because most talar OCDs are posteromedial, a plantar flexion AP and mortise view of the ankle puts the posterior talus in tangent, which improves OCD lesion visualization. This is similar to how the notch or tunnel view highlights a knee posterior condyle OCD lesion. Plain films may reveal other pathologic conditions, such as fractures, arthrosis, exostoses, and neoplasm. A classification that has withstood the test of time is that of Berndt and Hardy (**Fig. 2**).[7] Osteochondral fractures or OCD lesions are not always visualized on plain films,[33] particularly stage I lesions (**Fig. 3**). These occult lesions are usually seen on MRI scans.

CT scans have shown that lesions are larger than can be appreciated on radiograph and CT scan can be useful in preoperative planning[39,40] in determining the size and depth of OCD lesions.[41] CT arthrography can be useful when subarticular cysts are present to evaluate if the cyst communicates with the joint (**Fig. 4**).[39] CT scans also help identify the amount of bone attached to the osteochondral lesion that may make it more amenable to compression screw fixation.

MRI is more frequently used in the diagnosis and staging of OCD lesions of the talus and is valuable in the identification of radiographically occult osteochondral fractures. This imaging modality can evaluate breaches in the articular cartilage, signal intensity changes of the subchondral bone, as well as loose bodies in the ankle joint.[42,43] Importantly, osteochondral dissecans lesions that are loose can sometimes be clearly identified by MRI. This is invaluable because most investigators would recommend early surgical reduction and fixation in cases such as these. For example, the orientation of the loose or free fragment, including those that are flipped or rotated, can often be better judged on an MRI.

Nelson and colleagues[43] performed a study to see if MRI could accurately predict the arthroscopic stage of ankle osteochondral lesions. Preoperative MRIs were reviewed by radiologists in blinded evaluations. Radiologists predicted the arthroscopic stage in 11 of 12 subject and MRI overstaged the lesion in one subjects.

Verhagen and colleagues[44] performed a study in more than 100 subjects that examined the sensitivity and specificity of arthroscopy, MRI, CT scan, radiograph, and

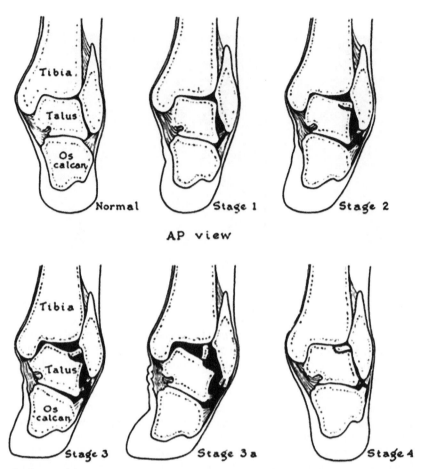

Fig. 2. Stage I lesions may not be visible on radiographs and are areas of subchondral compression. Stage II lesions are partially detached fragments of osteochondral fracture. Stage III lesions are nondisplaced fractures in which the osteochondral fragment is completely detached. Stage IV lesions are completely displaced loose bodies.[7] Later, Scranton added stage V for osteochondral lesions associated with a subchondral bone cyst.[83] (*From* Bernd AL, Harty M. Transchondral fractures (osteochondritis dissecans) of the talus. J Bone Joint Surg Am 1959;41-A:1002; with permission.)

physical examination for the detection of osteochondral lesions. Diagnostic arthroscopy demonstrated a sensitivity of 1 and specificity of 0.97. MRI without contrast resulted in 0.96 sensitivity and specificity. CT scans had a sensitivity and specificity of 0.81 and 0.99. Mortise view radiographs demonstrated sensitivity and specificity of 0.7 and 0.94, whereas history and physical examination was least sensitive (0.59) and specific (0.91).

NONOPERATIVE TREATMENT

In most cases, a trial of nonoperative treatment is pursued. Several studies have reported successful outcomes of nonoperative treatment of OLT,[41,45] even if radiographic evidence of the lesion persists.[36]

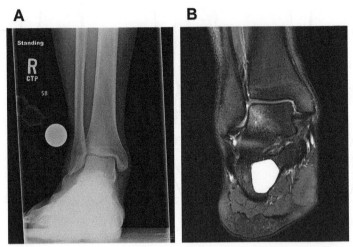

Fig. 3. (*A*) Plain mortise radiograph of a stage I lesion. (*B*) Coronal T2 MRI image of a stage I lesion.

Younger subjects have better healing potential than adults do. Lam and Siow's[45] study of six subjects with an average age of 12.3 (range 10.8–14.1) years who were followed for a mean of 30.5 months showed that all subjects had resolution of pain after 7 months. Five subjects had a good outcome and one had an excellent outcome. All subjects had some degree of radiographic healing and two had complete healing on radiographs.

Higuera and colleagues[41] reported on 18 subjects with an average age of 12.5 years. The mean time between onset of symptoms and diagnosis was 4.3 months and 10 subjects reported previous trauma to the ankle. Initially, subjects were treated with a cast and were non–weight bearing for 6 weeks. Subjects were followed for an additional 3.5 months with a structured program and progression of motion and strengthening with a high degree of success. A quarter of these subjects did not resolve their symptoms and underwent surgical intervention. They investigators did not report the results of nonoperative and operative treatment separately.

Letts and colleagues[37] performed a retrospective study of 24 children who were an average age of 13 years and an average follow-up of 16 months. Twenty-four subjects

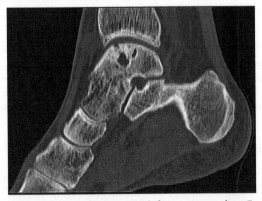

Fig. 4. CT scan of a patient with multiple cystic defects greater than 5 mm in depth.

were initially treated nonoperatively with activity and/or plaster immobilization in a walking cast for 5 weeks. Thirteen subjects failed nonoperative treatment due to persistent painful lesions and underwent subsequent operation.

Perumal and colleagues[36] performed a retrospective review of 31 subjects with a mean age of 11.9 years treated nonoperatively for OLT. Subjects were placed into a weight-bearing cast for 6 to 8 weeks and, after cast removal, a lace-up brace was applied. Sports, as well as running and jumping, was restricted for 6 months. Radiographs were taken at the end of 6 months and an MRI was performed if there were no radiographic signs of healing. If MRI demonstrated no signs of reossification and the subject was experiencing continued painful symptoms, surgical treatment was recommended. Subjects who were symptom free but had persistent unhealed osteochondral lesions on radiographs were offered the choice between surgery or nonoperative activity restriction and observation. After 6 months of nonoperative management, 16% of subjects had complete clinical and radiological improvement, whereas 77% had persistent radiographic lesions. The subjects with persistent OCD lesions underwent another 6 months of activity modification and 46% of these had no symptoms, despite persistent lesions on radiographs, and 42% of these underwent subsequent surgery for unhealed painful lesions.

McCullough and Venugopal[18] followed six subjects with a mean age of 27 years and a mean follow-up of 15 years, 11 months, who had medial OLT. Radiographically, five subjects had unhealed lesions and one was healed. Of the unhealed lesions, four reported good to excellent outcomes and one had a fair outcome. Only one of the unhealed lesions progressed to arthrosis and the investigators recommended that initial treatment should be cast immobilization for 2 months. Surgical intervention should be pursued if patients continue to have mechanical symptoms after 2 months.

For an average of 38 months, Shearer and colleagues[46] followed 34 subjects with stage V lesions who were managed nonoperatively. Only 54% of subjects had a good or excellent outcomes and 29% reported poor outcomes. Radiographically, most lesions remained stable and did not progress to arthrosis.

OPERATIVE TREATMENT

Indications for operative treatment of talar OCD lesions include radiographic evidence of an osteochondral lesion along with symptoms attributable to lesion, failure of conservative therapy in stage II and III lesions, and more immediate surgery in stage IV lesions.[47] Moreover, acute fractures of the talus, even those with minimal displacement, may do better with early reduction and fixation. Arthroscopy is now commonly used to treat osteochondral lesions and minimizes soft tissue trauma. Moreover, it can avoid potential complications such as nonunion from osteotomy[10] along with providing diminished morbidity and hospital time.[47] However, arthrotomies are still used in certain situations. In the past, some investigators thought that, due to small joint space in children, arthroscopes may be too large and the surgeon may have to perform an arthrotomy to access the talar dome.[37] Newer small joint arthroscopes with appropriate ankle distraction allow for safe arthroscopic examination of the ankle in smaller children. Posteromedial lesions that require internal fixation may be safely accessed via a 2 cm posteromedial approach with the patient held in forced dorsiflexion splitting between the tibialis posterior and flexor digitorum longus tendons.

Fragment Excision

O'Farrell and Costello[33] published a series of 24 subjects with 47 months of follow-up in which an arthrotomy was made to excise the osteochondral lesion. Fifteen subjects had good results, 9 fair, and there were no poor results. Lateral lesions were approached anteriorly and medial lesions used a medial malleolar osteotomy. One of 13 subjects with a medial malleolar osteotomy had a nonunion.

Bone Marrow Stimulation

The goal of bone marrow stimulation is to induce an inflammatory response to encourage healing of the subchondral lesion and to induce fibrocartilage formation in articular cartilage defects. Studies have indicated that this treatment strategy is an acceptable approach in lesions less than 15 mm in diameter.[48–53] Two common approaches to bone marrow stimulation have been described. Kumai and colleagues[54] reported a series of 18 ankles that underwent arthroscopy and transarticular drilling of the osteochondral lesion. Average subject age was 28 years and they were followed for a mean of 4.6 years. Osteochondral lesions were probed and the cartilaginous surface was found to be softened compared with the neighboring healthy articular cartilage. A 1 or 1.2 mm Kirschner (k-) wire was passed through the articular surface to stimulate bleeding from the subchondral bone. Overall, all ankles improved after treatment and 13 subjects achieved a good result, whereas five subjects had a fair result. Twelve of 13 ankles that were under age 30 at the time of operation had good results in contrast to one in five ankles in subjects over age 50.

Similar to avascular necrosis lesions in the femoral head, the goal in retrograde drilling is to preserve articular cartilage and revitalize subchondral bone. Taranow and colleagues[55] described a technique of retrograde drilling of medial osteochondral lesions with an intact cartilage surface. A guidewire was drilled through the sinus tarsi into the base of the osteochondral lesion. A 3.5 to 4.5 mm cannulated drill was passed up the guidewire to the base of the lesion without violating the articular surface. A graft was then harvested from the ipsilateral calcaneus using a Craig needle and injected into the drill path. This was performed in 16 ankles and followed for an average of 2 months. American Orthopaedic Foot and Ankle Society (AOFAS) Ankle-Hindfoot scores improved from 53.9 to 82.6 at follow-up. Overall satisfaction was 81% and mean time to radiographic healing was 7 months; 88% of subjects had radiographic healing (**Fig. 5**).

Anders and colleagues[56] reported a series of 41 lesions in 38 subjects who underwent fluoroscopic retrograde drilling and autologous bone grafting. Subjects had a mean follow-up of 29 months. AOFAS scores improved from 47.3 to 80.8. Grade I and II lesions improved more than grade III lesions, suggesting that retrograde drilling is the preferred method of treating lesions with intact cartilage.

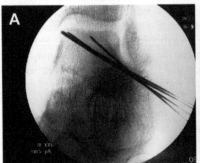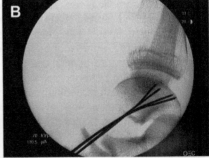

Fig. 5. (A, B) Coronal and sagittal fluoroscopy images during arthroscopically aided percutaneous retrograde drilling of a 14-year-old female with a medial talar OCD lesion.

Microfracture

Microfracture involves excising the cartilage defect and inducing bleeding from the subchondral bone. This allows mesenchymal stem cells to be brought to the defect. The defect then heals with a fibrocartilage scar.[57] This may be performed either arthroscopically or through an arthrotomy and, sometimes, a medial malleolar osteotomy for medial lesions. This is in contrast to transarticular drilling in which the lesion is kept in situ and drilling through the lesion is done to stimulate healing of the progeny lesion.

Chuckpaiwong and colleagues[49] reported a series of 105 osteochondral lesions treated with microfracture and a mean follow-up of 12.1 months. There were no treatment failures in lesions smaller than 15 mm and only one success in lesions greater than 15 mm. Other factors that were associated with treatment failure were age, higher body mass index, trauma, and arthrosis.

Alexander and Lichtman[8] followed 35 subjects for 65 months who underwent curettage and drilling of an osteochondral lesion of the talus. Subjects were rated as excellent if they could run without pain, good if they could walk without pain but had pain with running, fair if they had slight restrictions with walking but did not require pain medication for normal activities, and poor if they required assistive devices for ambulation or underwent subsequent surgeries. Twenty-two subjects had good or excellent results.

Flick and Gould[30] performed a retrospective study in 22 subjects with an average follow-up of 24 months. Lateral lesions were approached via an anterolateral approach and medial lesions were approached through the anterior tibialis tendon sheath. Seventy nine percents of subjects had good or excellent results, two fair, and no poor results.

Ferkel and Chams[10] performed a retrospective study of 50 subjects who had failed at least 4 months of nonoperative treatment. The average age of the subjects was 32 years and average follow-up time was 71 months. Six subjects underwent excision of the lesion and abrasion arthroplasty and 40 subjects underwent excision and drilling of the lesion. Seventy two percent of subjects achieved good to excellent results, 20% fair, and 6% had poor results.

Becher and Thermann[58] performed a prospective study in 30 subjects with an average age of 41 years who were treated with arthroscopic microfracture. Mean follow-up was 2 years and 83% of subjects had good or excellent outcomes. Subjects older than the age of 50 did not have inferior results compared with younger subjects.

Gobbi and colleagues[59] performed a randomized controlled trial comparing chondroplasty, microfracture, and osteochondral autograft transplantation in 33 ankles with 53 month follow-up. Eleven subjects underwent chondroplasty, 10 had microfracture, and 12 underwent osteochondral autograft transplantation. All subjects demonstrated statistically significant improvement in all treatment groups and there were no significant differences between the groups.

Van Buecken and colleagues[47] performed a retrospective review of 15 cases of OLTs treated with arthroscopic subchondral drilling. Minimum time to follow-up was 18 months and average age of subjects was 22.6 years. At final follow-up, nine subjects had excellent results, four good, one fair, and one poor. Seven of 15 lesions demonstrated evidence of bony healing on radiographs but these subjects had equivalent clinical results to those who had unhealed lesions.

Lee and colleagues[60] reported a series of subjects less than 50 years old (average age 35) with lesions smaller than 15 mm who underwent arthroscopic microfracture. Mean follow-up time was 33 months. 89% of subjects had good-to-excellent results according to the AOFAS score. Mean AOFAS score improved from 63 points preoperatively to 90 points postoperatively.

Schuman and colleagues[61] reported a series of 38 subjects with a minimum follow-up of 2 years who were treated with arthroscopic curettage and drilling. Average age of subjects was 29.3 years and mean time to follow-up was 4.8 years. Good to excellent results were achieved in 82% of subjects.

Cuttica and colleagues[62] performed a study using MRI to evaluate edema and healing following arthroscopic microfracture of OLTs. MRIs were performed at a minimum of 9 months following surgery and studies were graded by a musculoskeletal radiologist. Thirty osteochondral lesions were included and the average age of subjects was 31.9 years. Subjects with moderate or severe edema had inferior clinical outcomes, whereas subjects with less edema had better outcomes.

Lee and colleagues[63] performed second look arthroscopies in 20 ankles at 12 months following arthroscopic microfracture of talar osteochondral lesions. Although seven of 20 ankles showed incomplete healing, 90% of ankles achieved excellent or good outcomes.

Osteochondral Autograft Transplantation

Osteochondral bone plugs using autograft can be used to replace the osteochondral lesions in the talar dome. Biopsies of these grafts at 2 years have shown that the grafted articular cartilage survived and fibrocartilage fills the space at the graft-lesion interface. Autologous grafts are typically harvested from the non–weight bearing areas of the distal femur. Marymont and colleagues[64] used MRI reconstructions to compare the articular morphology of the distal femur with the talus and found that the superolateral femur was the most congruous donor site for both medial and lateral talar lesions.

Larger lesions may require multiple bone plugs to reconstruct the articular surface of the talus. Choung and Christensen[65] performed a cadaveric study to determine whether repairing large osteochondral lesions in the talar dome can restore ankle joint surface mechanics. Using pressure sensitive film, they showed that contact pressures could be restored and that using multiple small grafts restored contact pressures better than fewer large grafts. In a later study, Hangody and colleagues[66] retrospectively reviewed 36 subjects at an average of 4.2 years following mosaicplasty using grafts from the ipsilateral knee. Lesions were stage III and IV and measured at least 10 mm. An average of three grafts was used to fill the defects and there was no long-term donor site morbidity. There was no radiographic subsidence of the grafts and 28 subjects had excellent outcomes, 6 good, and 2 moderate.

Al-Shaikh and colleagues[67] reported on 19 subjects with an average age of 32 with an average of 16 months follow-up. Donor plugs were harvested from the superolateral aspect of the lateral femoral condyle of the distal femur. Medial malleolar osteotomy was performed in 13 subjects and there were no nonunions of the osteotomies. There were two superficial neuromas and one subject with symptomatic hardware from the osteotomy.

Sammarco and Makwana[68] used local osteochondral autografts to avoid donor site morbidity in the knee. Grafts were harvested from the distal anterior surface of the talar dome and placed into the defect. AOFAS scores improved from 64.4 preoperatively to 90.8 at 25.3 months after surgery. There were no complications from the donor site.

Kumai and colleagues[69] reported on 27 subjects with an average age of 27.8 and mean follow-up of 7 years. Grafts were harvested from the ipsilateral distal tibia articular surface. Results were good in 24 subjects and fair in 3. Full range of motion was achieved in 22 subjects and 13 subjects returned to sporting activity. There were no complications. Bony union on either CT scan or radiograph was rated as good if there was complete bony union, fair if there was incomplete bony union, and poor if there was no change or collapse of the grafts. Twenty-two subjects were rated as good, two as fair, and three as poor radiographically.

Emre and colleagues[70] reported 2-year outcomes in a prospective study of 32 subjects who were treated with mosaicplasty harvested from the ipsilateral knee. The mean size of the lesions was 1.13 cm^2 and the AOFAS scores improved from 59.12 to 87.94 postoperatively. There were no infections, bleeding complications, or reoperations and donor site pain resolved in all subjects by 6 months postoperatively.

Lee and colleagues[71] reported a series of 18 subjects with an average age of 22.7 and a mean follow-up period of 36 months. Eleven of the 18 subjects had stage IV and 7 had stage III lesions. Two to three plugs measuring 6 or 7 mm were used and 16 subjects had excellent results and two reported good results. Thirteen subjects were able to return to sports and six of those were at preinjury levels. Fifteen subjects reported mild soreness with knee flexion at the time of follow-up.

Osteochondral Allograft Transplantation

When OLTs are too large, osteochondral allograft transplants have been used to replace the osteochondral lesion.[72–74] Osteochondral allografts hold the advantage of being able to reconstruct both the superior and the vertical surfaces involved in most OLTs with articular cartilage.

Gross and colleagues[73] reported a series of nine subjects with a mean age of 38 years on medial talar lesions of at least 1 cm diameter and 5 mm in depth in which the fragment could not be reattached. A medial malleolar osteotomy was performed and the talar lesion was debrided. The edges of the defect were cut squarely to accept a size-matched talar allograft that had been harvested within 24 to 48 hours before surgery. Internal fixation was achieved using one or two countersunk mini-fragment cancellous screws. Nine stage IV lesions were followed for 12 years and three of these subjects had subsequent ankle arthrodesis at the time of follow-up. Six of the surviving grafts were able to walk without any assistive devices, five of which had no residual ankle pain and one subject had minor limitations with recreational activity. Of the three subjects who needed subsequent ankle fusion, all had radiographic evidence of graft fragmentation and partial resorption. There were no signs of immunologic graft rejection (**Fig. 6**).

Raikin[74] reported a series of subjects with large osteochondral defects measuring greater than 3 cm diameter with an average volume of 4.38 cm^3 in six subjects. There were five medial and one lateral lesion. The defect in the talus was excised and the transplanted osteochondral graft was placed and fixed using headless compression screws. The average preoperative AOFAS score was 42 and it improved to 86 at the 2-year follow-up.

Chondrocyte Implantation

Cartilage implantation is a treatment modality that consists of harvesting healthy chondrocytes, culturing the cells, and performing a second procedure in which the chondrocytes are implanted into the defect.

Koulalis and colleagues[75,76] performed autologous chondrocyte transplant in 8 subjects with an average age of 31.8 and a follow-up of 17.6 months. Lesion size ranged from approximately 10mm^2 to 25mm^2. Subjects underwent an initial ankle arthroscopy and a cartilage biopsy was performed. The chondrocytes were sent to a laboratory and cultured. Two and a half weeks later, a second procedure was performed and a medial malleolar osteotomy was performed to access the talar dome lesion. The osteochondral lesion was debrided and a periosteal flap from the anterior tibia was sewn over the defect using 5-0 polydioxanone suture. The chondrocytes were then implanted under the periosteal flap and the subjects were made non–weight bearing

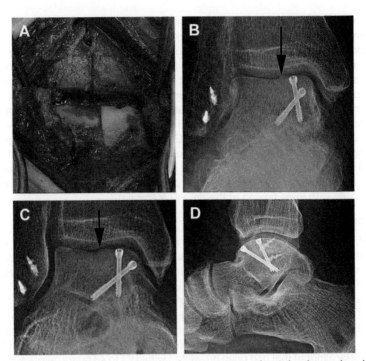

Fig. 6. Intraoperative appearance of the graft demonstrates that it has been placed flush to native cartilage. (*A*) Radiographic appearance at 1 year demonstrates incorporation of the graft; however, note the elevated of appearance of the subchondral bone (*arrow*) on the AP (*B*) and mortise (*C*) radiographs. The asymmetric appearance can be difficult to view on the lateral radiograph (*D*).

for 6 to 7 weeks but were permitted to perform range of motion exercises. MRI was performed at 3, 6, and 12 months postoperatively. These MRIs did not show evidence of cartilage incorporation until the 12 month MRI. Five subjects reported an excellent outcome and three subjects reported very good results.

Schneider and Karaikudi[77] reported on 20 subjects with an average age of 36 who underwent matrix-induced autologous chondrocyte implantation. Mean lesion size was 232.7 mm^2 (range 63–630 mm^2). The chondrocytes were cultured onto a porcine collagen membrane and this membrane was placed onto the OCD lesion and secured using fibrin glue. Subjects were non–weight bearing for 6 weeks and the investigators permitted range of motion exercises after the wound was healed. Average AOFAS scores improved from 60 preoperatively to 86.9 postoperatively. Five subjects underwent subsequent removal of hardware from a medial malleolar osteotomy and two subjects had failed grafts.

Anders and colleagues[78] reported on 22 subjects treated with matrix-associated autologous chondrocyte implantation. The average age of subjects was 23.9 and they were followed for a mean of 63.5 months. The average size of the osteochondral defects was 1.94 cm^2. Average AOFAS scores improved from 70.1 to 95.3 and there were no reported complications.

Complications

The reported complication rate in ankle arthroscopy is about 10%.[79] Most are found to largely consist of transient neurologic injury.[80] Other complications include superficial infection, synovial fistulas, portal pain, and vascular and cartilage damage.[80–82] Gobbi and colleagues[59] compared arthroscopic chondroplasty versus microfracture versus osteochondral autologous transplantation, noting persistent pain as the only complication in each of the three groups. Finally, complications for open arthrotomy and debridement of OCD lesions are notable for malleolus nonunion in 12.5% following medial malleolus osteotomy for access to posterior talus lesions.[8,33]

AUTHORS' PREFERRED TECHNIQUE

The authors recommend appropriately matching to the simplest technique that has a reasonable rate of healing clinically and generating a good or excellent outcome. Patients who present with asymptomatic OLTs on radiographs taken for other reasons (eg, for a lateral ankle sprain) do not need treatment. For patients who present with a painful OLT, we recommend non–weight bearing immobilization, with a cast or controlled ankle motion (CAM) walker boot, for about 6 weeks. We then switch to a brace for about 6 more weeks and start rehabilitation to regain motion and strength and stability of the ankle. If the ankle pain resolves, we allow return to full activity and sports when cleared by a therapist or a trainer, even if there is no resolution on x-rays. If pain persists after immobilization and rehabilitation, we obtain an MRI scan to size, locate, and stage the lesion. Perilesional edema seen on MRI strongly suggests that the patient's OLT is the cause of their ankle pain.

Patients failing nonoperative management are recommended to have an arthroscopic evaluation with a 2.7 mm arthroscope. If the lesion's articular cartilage is intact on all articular surfaces, including the vertical surface in the gutter, and the cartilage has normal consistency to probing, then retroarticular drilling with bone grafting (using the methods of Taranow and colleagues[55] and Anders and colleagues[56]) are preferred.

If the articular surface is breeched, but the cartilage is normal in appearance and consistency, then internal fixation may be indicated through either an arthroscopic or an open approach. This is best indicated when the OLT lesion has a substantial bone attached to the articular cartilage. Most OCD lesions that are posteromedial may be accessed via a 2 cm skin incision just posterior to medial malleolus. Dissection proceeds between the tibialis posterior and flexor digitorum longus. This provides easy access to the posteromedial talus that is well exposed with 90° knee flexion and maximum ankle dorsiflexion.

OLTs that are less than 1.5 cm and have soft or degenerated cartilage are probably best treated with curettage and debridement, followed by marrow stimulation with drill, k-wire, or pick penetration to normal talar bone. The authors use microcurettes, both angled and straight, and ENT stapes curettes. These curettes must be extremely sharp to make a clean vertical wall of the crater. A 2.5 or 3.5 mm full radius (toothless) shaver is used to clean out small debris. Hand traction with a foot strap helps to open up the joint to avoid any iatrogenic damage to the normal tibial, fibular, or talar cartilage. Postoperatively, the authors recommend aggressive range of motion, but non–weight bearing, for 6 weeks, followed by transition to full weight bearing over the next 2 weeks. Return to sports is allowed at 4 to 6 months postoperatively depending on the patient's pain free lower extremity strength, motion, stability, and agility.

Talar lesions that are greater than 1.5 cm in diameter but less than 4 cm^2 surface area may do best with osteochondral autograft transplantation. These lesions are most commonly located on the medial talus and often require a medial malleolus osteotomy. These osteotomies can be complicated by malunion or nonunion. The authors recommend starting the osteotomy with multiple drill holes along the osteotomy plane, using a sagittal saw with a very thin blade about halfway to the joint, and then completing the osteotomy with a thin and sharp Hoke osteotome. Before completing the osteotomy, it is best to drill two transverse pilot holes for dual screw fixation. Before completing the osteotomy, one can temporarily place the screws to make screw tracks, then remove the screws and complete the osteotomy with the thin osteotomes. This will help with anatomic fixation of the osteotomy during closure.

Fresh osteochondral allograft transplantation is best indicated for the largest talar OLTs, especially those that involve the medial or lateral walls of the talar dome. Generally, the patient's talar defect is exposed via a malleolar osteotomy and a quadrilateral segment containing the OLT is removed and replaced with a matching quadrilateral portion of similar sized donor talus.

SUMMARY

OCDs and OLTs are relatively uncommon sources of ankle pain in adolescents and adults that are not always apparent on ankle radiographs. OLTs have been associated with acute ankle trauma but the exact cause of OCD of the talus, as with other joints, remains elusive. These are often radiographically occult and can cause late ankle pain. MRI illuminates the location, stage, and displacement of the talar lesions, and it should be considered when pain persists after nonoperative treatment. Immobilization and activity limitation for 6 to 12 weeks is the first line treatment of symptomatic lesions. Failing this, retroarticular drilling with or without bone grafting is indicated for intact lesions with pristine articular cartilage. Nondisplaced lesions with an articular fissure or demarcation may do well with compression screw repair especially if the cartilage is attached to subchondral bone. Lesions without pristine articular cartilage that are less than 15 mm long do well with fragment excision and marrow stimulation. Larger lesions with poor articular cartilage can be treated with osteochondral autograft, fresh osteochondral allograft, or chondrocyte regeneration techniques with high success. Outcomes after OCD surgical treatment often yield 70% to 90% good or excellent results, with the level of surgery matched to the stage and state of the OCD or OLT lesion.

REFERENCES

1. Monro A. Part of the cartilage of the joint separated and ossified. Medical Essays Observations 1738;4:19.
2. Konig F. The classic: on loose bodies in the joint. 1887. Clin Orthop Relat Res 2013;471(4):1107–15.
3. Kappis M. Weitere beitrage zur traumatisch-mechanischen entstehung der "spontanen" knorpela biosungen. Deutsche Zeitschrift für Chirurgie (in German) 1922;171:13–29.
4. Research in osteochondritis dissecans of the knee (ROCK). Available at: http://kneeocd.org. Accessed January 24, 2014.
5. Edmonds EW, Shea KG. Osteochondritis dissecans: editorial comment. Clin Orthop Relat Res 2013;471(4):1105–6.
6. Orr JD, Dawson LK, Garcia EJ, et al. Incidence of osteochondral lesions of the talus in the United States military. Foot Ankle Int 2011;32:948–54.
7. Berndt AL, Harty M. Osteochondritis dissecans of the ankle joint; report of a case simulating a fracture of the talus. J Bone Joint Surg Am 1959;41-A:988–1020.
8. Alexander AH, Lichtman DM. Surgical treatment of transchondral talar-dome fractures (osteochondritis dissecans). Long-term follow-up. J Bone Joint Surg Am 1980;62(4):646–52.

9. Draper SD, Fallat LM. Autogenous bone grafting for the treatment of talar dome lesions. J Foot Ankle Surg 2000;39:15–23.

10. Ferkel RD, Chams RN. Chronic lateral instability: arthroscopic findings and long-term results. Foot Ankle Int 2007;28(1):24–31.

11. Leontaritis N, Hinojosa L, Panchbhavi VK. Arthroscopically detected intra-articular lesions associated with acute ankle fractures. J Bone Joint Surg Am 2009;91:333–9.

12. Sneppen O, Christensen SB, Krogsoe O, et al. Fracture of the body of the talus. Acta Orthop Scand 1977;48:317–24.

13. Elias I, Zoga AC, Morrison WB, et al. Osteochondral lesions of the talus: local-ization and morphologic data from 424 patients using a novel anatomical grid scheme. Foot Ankle Int 2007;28(2):154–61.

14. Hembree WC, Wittstein JR, Vinson EN, et al. Magnetic resonance imaging fea-tures of osteochondral lesions of the talus. Foot Ankle Int 2012;33(7):591–7.

15. Ray RB, Coughlin EJ Jr. Osteochondritis dissecans of the talus. J Bone Joint Surg Am 1947;29:697–706.

16. Marks KL. Osteochondritis dissecans of the talus in recurrent ankle sprains. J Bone Joint Surg Br 1952;34-B:90–2.

17. Cameron BM. Osteochondritis dissecans of the talus. J Bone Joint Surg Am 1956;38-A:857–61.

18. McCullough CJ, Venugopal V. Osteochondritis dissecans of the talus: the natu-ral history. Clin Orthop Relat Res 1979;(144):264–8.

19. Anderson DV, Lyne ED. Osteochondritis dissecans of the talus: case report on two family members. J Pediatr Orthop 1984;4:356–7.

20. Woods K, Harris I. Osteochondritis dissecans of the talus in identical twins. J Bone Joint Surg Br 1995;77:331.

21. Hammett RB, Saxby TS. Osteochondral lesion of the talus in homozygous twins–the question of heredity. Foot Ankle Surg 2010;16(3):e55–6.

22. Mandracchia VJ, Buddecke DE, Giesking JL. Osteochondral lesions of the talar dome. A comprehensive review with retrospective study. Clin Podiatr Med Surg 1999;16:725–42.

23. Giannini S, Buda R, Faldini C, et al. Surgical treatment of osteochondral lesions of the talus in young active patients. J Bone Joint Surg Am 2005;87(Suppl 2):28–41.

24. Thompson JP, Loomer RL. Osteochondral lesions of the talus in a sports med-icine clinic. A new radiographic technique and surgical approach. Am J Sports Med 1984;12:460–3.

25. Tol JL, Struijs PA, Bossuyt PM, et al. Treatment strategies in osteochondral de-fects of the talar dome: a systematic review. Foot Ankle Int 2000;21:119–26.

26. DIGiovanni BF, Fraga CJ, Cohen BE, et al. Associated injuries found in chronic lateral ankle instability. Foot Ankle Int 2000;21(10):809–15.

27. Koch S, Kampen WU, Laprell H. Cartilage and bone morphology in osteochon-dritis dissecans. Knee Surg Sports Traumatol Arthrosc 1997;5:42–5.

28. Canale ST, Belding RH. Osteochondral lesions of the talus. J Bone Joint Surg Am 1980;62:97–102.

29. Canale ST, Kelly FB. Fractures of the neck of the talus. Long-term evaluation of seventy-one cases. J Bone Joint Surg Am 1978;60:143–56.

30. Flick AB, Gould N. Osteochondritis dissecans of the talus (transchondral frac-tures of the talus): review of the literature and new surgical approach for medial dome lesions. Foot Ankle 1985;5:165–85.

31. Robinson DE, Winson IG, Harries WJ, et al. Arthroscopic treatment of osteo-chondral lesions of the talus. J Bone Joint Surg Br 2003;85(7):989–93.

32. Bruns J, Rosenbach B. Osteochondrosis dissecans of the talus. Comparison of results of surgical treatment in adolescents and adults. Arch Orthop Trauma Surg 1992;112:23–7.

33. O'Farrell TA, Costello BG. Osteochondritis dissecans of the talus. The late results of surgical treatment. J Bone Joint Surg Br 1982;64:494–7.

34. Roden S, Tillegard P, Unanderscharin L. Flake fracture of the talus progressing to osteochondritis dissecans. Acta Orthop Scand 1953;23:51–66.

35. Loomer R, Fisher C, Lloyd-Smith R, et al. Osteochondral lesions of the talus. Am J Sports Med 1993;21(1):13–9.

36. Perumal V, Wall E, Babekir N. Juvenile osteochondritis dissecans of the talus. J Pediatr Orthop 2007;27:821–5.

37. Letts M, Davidson D, Ahmer A. Osteochondritis dissecans of the talus in children. J Pediatr Orthop 2003;23:617–25.

38. Haskell A, Mann R. In: DeLee J, Drez D, Miller MD, editors. DeLee & Drez's orthopaedic sports medicine: principles and practice. Philadelphia: Saunders/Elsevier; 2009. p. 2144.

39. Davies AM, Cassar-Pullicino V. Demonstration of osteochondritis dissecans of the talus by coronal computed tomographic arthrography. Br J Radiol 1989;62:1050.

40. Zinman C, Wolfson N, Reis ND. Osteochondritis dissecans of the dome of the talus. Computed tomography scanning in diagnosis and follow-up. J Bone Joint Surg Am 1988;70:1017–9.

41. Higuera J, Laguna R, Peral M, et al. Osteochondritis dissecans of the talus during childhood and adolescence. J Pediatr Orthop 1998;18:328.

42. De Smet AA, Fisher DR, Burnstein MI, et al. Value of MR imaging in staging osteochondral lesions of the talus (osteochondritis dissecans): results in 14 patients. AJR Am J Roentgenol 1990;154:555–8.

43. Nelson DW, DiPaola J, Colville M, et al. Osteochondritis dissecans of the talus and knee: prospective comparison of MR and arthroscopic classifications. J Comput Assist Tomogr 1990;14:804–8.

44. Verhagen RA, Struijs PA, Bossuyt PM, et al. Systematic review of treatment strategies for osteochondral defects of the talar dome. Foot Ankle Clin 2003;8:233–42.

45. Lam KY, Siow HM. Conservative treatment for juvenile osteochondritis dissecans of the talus. J Orthop Surg (Hong Kong) 2012;20:176–80.

46. Shearer C, Loomer R, Clement D. Nonoperatively managed stage 5 osteochondral talar lesions. Foot Ankle Int 2002;23:651–4.

47. Van Buecken K, Barrack RL, Alexander AH, et al. Arthroscopic treatment of transchondral talar dome fractures. Am J Sports Med 1989;17:350–5 [discussion: 355–6].

48. Amendola A, Panarella L. Osteochondral lesions: medial versus lateral, persistent pain, cartilage restoration options and indications. Foot Ankle Clin 2009;14:215–27.

49. Chuckpaiwong B, Berkson EM, Theodore GH. Microfracture for osteochondral lesions of the ankle: outcome analysis and outcome predictors of 105 cases. Arthroscopy 2008;24:106–12.

50. Giannini S, Vannini F. Operative treatment of osteochondral lesions of the talar dome: current concepts review. Foot Ankle Int 2004;25:168–75.

51. van Dijk CN, van Bergen CJ. Advancements in ankle arthroscopy. J Am Acad Orthop Surg 2008;16:635–46.

52. Lahm A, Erggelet C, Steinwachs M, et al. Arthroscopic management of osteochondral lesions of the talus: results of drilling and usefulness of magnetic resonance imaging before and after treatment. Arthroscopy 2000;16:299–304.

53. Zengerink M, Struijs PA, Tol JL, et al. PMC2809940; Treatment of osteochondral lesions of the talus: a systematic review. Knee Surg Sports Traumatol Arthrosc 2010;18:238–46.

54. Kumai T, Takakura Y, Higashiyama I, et al. Arthroscopic drilling for the treatment of osteochondral lesions of the talus. J Bone Joint Surg Am 1999;81:1229–35.

55. Taranow WS, Bisignani GA, Towers JD, et al. Retrograde drilling of osteochondral lesions of the medial talar dome. Foot Ankle Int 1999;20:474–80.

56. Anders S, Lechler P, Rackl W, et al. Fluoroscopy-guided retrograde core drilling and cancellous bone grafting in osteochondral defects of the talus. Int Orthop 2012;36(8):1635–40.

57. Steadman JR, Rodkey WG, Rodrigo JJ. Microfracture: surgical technique and rehabilitation to treat chondral defects. Clin Orthop Relat Res 2001;(Suppl 391):S362–9.

58. Becher C, Thermann H. Results of microfracture in the treatment of articular cartilage defects of the talus. Foot Ankle Int 2005;26(8):583–9.

59. Gobbi A, Francisco RA, Lubowitz JH, et al. Osteochondral lesions of the talus: randomized controlled trial comparing chondroplasty, microfracture, and osteochondral autograft transplantation. Arthroscopy 2006;22(10):1085–92.

60. Lee KB, Bai LB, Chung JY, et al. Arthroscopic microfracture for osteochondral lesions of the talus. Knee Surg Sports Traumatol Arthrosc 2010;18:247–53. http://dx.doi.org/10.1007/s00167-009-0914-x.

61. Schuman L, Struijs PA, van Dijk CN. Treatment of cartilage defects of the talus by autologous osteochondral grafts. J Bone Joint Surg Br 2002;84:364–8.

62. Cuttica DJ, Shockley JA, Hyer CF, et al. Correlation of MRI edema and clinical outcomes following microfracture of osteochondral lesions of the talus. Foot Ankle Spec 2011;4:274–9. http://dx.doi.org/10.1177/1938640011411082.

63. Lee KB, Bai LB, Yoon TR, et al. Second-look arthroscopic findings and clinical outcomes after microfracture for osteochondral lesions of the talus. Am J Sports Med 2009;37:63S–70S. http://dx.doi.org/10.1177/0363546509348471.

64. Marymont JV, Shute G, Zhu H, et al. Computerized matching of autologous femoral grafts for the treatment of medial talar osteochondral defects. Foot Ankle Int 2005;26:708–12.

65. Choung D, Christensen JC. Mosaicplasty of the talus: a joint contact analysis in a cadaver model. J Foot Ankle Surg 2002;41:65–75.

66. Hangody L, Kish G, Modis L, et al. Mosaicplasty for the treatment of osteochondritis dissecans of the talus: two to seven year results in 36 patients. Foot Ankle Int 2001;22:552–8.

67. Al-Shaikh R, Chou LB, Mann JA, et al. Autologous osteochondral grafting for talar cartilage defects. Foot Ankle Int 2002;23:381–9.

68. Sammarco GJ, Makwana NK. Treatment of talar osteochondral lesions using local osteochondral graft. Foot Ankle Int 2002;23:693–8.

69. Kumai T, Takakura Y, Kitada C, et al. Fixation of osteochondral lesions of the talus using cortical bone pegs. J Bone Joint Surg Br 2002;84(3):369–74.

70. Emre TY, Ege T, Cift HT, et al. Open mosaicplasty in osteochondral lesions of the talus: a prospective study. J Foot Ankle Surg 2012;51:556–60. http://dx.doi.org/10.1053/j.jfas.2012.05.006.

71. Lee CH, Chao KH, Huang GS, et al. Osteochondral autografts for osteochondritis dissecans of the talus. Foot Ankle Int 2003;24:815–22.

72. Lee CK, Mercurio C. Operative treatment of osteochondritis dissecans in situ by retrograde drilling and cancellous bone graft: a preliminary report. Clin Orthop Relat Res 1981;158. p. 129–36.

73. Gross AE, Agnidis Z, Hutchison CR. Treatment of type V osteochondral lesions of the talus with ipsilateral knee osteochondral autografts. Foot Ankle Int 2001; 22:385–91.

74. Raikin SM. Stage VI: massive osteochondral defects of the talus. Foot Ankle Clin 2004;9:737–44.

75. Koulalis D, Schultz W, Psychogios B, et al. Articular reconstruction of osteochondral defects of the talus through autologous chondrocyte transplantation. Orthopedics 2004;27:559–61.

76. Koulalis D, Schultz W, Heyden M. Autologous chondrocyte transplantation for osteochondritis dissecans of the talus. Clin Orthop Relat Res 2002;186–92.

77. Schneider TE, Karaikudi S. Matrix-Induced Autologous Chondrocyte Implantation (MACI) grafting for osteochondral lesions of the talus. Foot Ankle Int 2009;30:810–4. http://dx.doi.org/10.3113/FAI.2009.0810.

78. Anders S, Goetz J, Schubert T, et al. Treatment of deep articular talus lesions by matrix associated autologous chondrocyte implantation–results at five years. Int Orthop 2012;36:2279–85. http://dx.doi.org/10.1007/s00264-012-1635-1.

79. Zengerink M, van Dijk CN. Complications in ankle arthroscopy. Knee Surg Sports Traumatol Arthrosc 2012;20(8):1420–31.

80. Carlson MJ, Ferkel RD. Complications in ankle and foot arthroscopy. Sports Med Arthrosc 2013;21(2):135–9.

81. Guhl JF. New concepts (distraction) in ankle arthroscopy. Arthroscopy 1988; 4(3):160–7.

82. Barber FA, Click J, Britt BT. Complications of ankle arthroscopy. Foot Ankle 1990;10(5):263–6.

83. Scranton PE Jr, McDermott JE. Treatment of type V osteochondral lesions of the talus with ipsilateral knee osteochondral autografts. Foot Ankle Int 2001;22: 380–4.

Osteochondritis Dissecans of the Shoulder and Hip

Eric W. Edmonds, MD[a,b,*], Benton E. Heyworth, MD[c]

KEYWORDS

- Osteochondritis dissecans • Shoulder • Hip

KEY POINTS

- Both osteochondritis dissecans (OCD) of the shoulder and hip are uncommon findings with shoulder OCD being more prevalent, accounting for 1.6% of OCDs found in children.
- Shoulder OCD may involve either the glenoid or the humeral head, and case reports suggest that humeral OCD responds well to drilling.
- Hip OCD may involve either the acetabulum or the femoral head, and either one may require major surgery to alleviate symptoms in this weight-bearing joint.
- There is a case report suggesting that acetabular OCDs may resolve without surgical intervention.
- Femoral head OCD may, in fact, be a sequela of Legg-Calve-Perthes disease or avascular necrosis of the hip in a focal form, or there may be overlap between the 3 pathologies.

INTRODUCTION

Osteochondritis dissecans (OCD) is a poorly understood disease of the articular cartilage and subchondral bone that was first described in 1887 as a cause of intra-articular loose bodies.[1,2] The most common location is the knee, followed by the ankle and elbow, but there is evidence that the pathologic process can involve the shoulder and hip joints.[1] The most recent definition of human OCD lesions, proposed by the Research in Osteochondritis of the Knee (ROCK) study group, highlights the fact that these are (1) focal, (2) idiopathic, (3) involve subchondral bone, and (4) risk instability and disruption of articular cartilage with potential long-term consequences, such as premature osteoarthritis.[3] Understanding of OCD in the comparative literature of veterinary medicine highlights the possibility that these lesions may actually originate

[a] Division of Orthopedic Surgery, Rady Children's Hospital and Health Center, 3030 Children's Way, Suite 410, San Diego, CA 92123, USA; [b] Department of Orthopedic Surgery, University of California San Diego, 200 West Arbor Drive, San Diego, CA 92103, USA; [c] Division of Sports Medicine, Department of Orthopedic Surgery, Boston Children's Hospital, Harvard Medical School, 300 Longwood Avenue, Boston, MA 02115, USA
* Corresponding author. 3030 Children's Way, Suite 410, San Diego, CA 92123.
E-mail address: ewedmonds@rchsd.org

within the cartilage anlage of the subchondral bone, and this concept needs to be considered when reviewing the literature on human shoulder and hip OCD.[4,5] Keeping a working definition in mind, as well as the etiologic theory of OCD origin in animals, a review of the literature for OCD of the shoulder and hip finds conflicting reports, of which, many may not be true OCD lesions.

SHOULDER OCD

A recent epidemiology study looking at the prevalence of OCD in the population at different anatomic sites found that shoulder OCD accounted for 1.6% of all OCD between the ages of 6 and 19 years, with an incidence of 0.3 cases per 100,000 population.[6] A search of PubMed using the keywords "osteochondritis dissecans shoulder" yielded 94 different publications in all languages when performed on July 10, 2013. Most of these publications were from veterinary medicine colleagues and involved the humeral head of both cats and dogs. The literature on people, however, demonstrated both humeral head and glenoid fossa involvement.

Humeral head OCD has been presented in 8 different publications since 1950 with 12 different cases being reported in the literature.[7–14] It seems that all of the case reports identify pain as at least one of the presenting symptoms, and no reports were identified incidentally. It seems that this alone may indicate that the development of a humeral head OCD may be secondary to microtrauma, an etiology proposed for this anatomic site by Mahirogullari and colleagues.[9] There may be a predilection for males (9 out of 12 cases), and there may be an age bias for the young, with 5 cases being 12 to 19 years old, with no cases found in the elderly population (in contrast to glenoid lesions).[9,11,14] Radiographic assessment by plain film yielded a radiolucent lesion with a sclerotic rim in most cases, specifically involving the anterosuperior aspect of the humeral head.[8,9,11] Likely, this sclerotic rim represents a pseudocortex forming adjacent the OCD, which is seen in other joint OCDs. Furthermore, magnetic resonance imaging (MRI) can confirm the diagnosis with an appearance that is believed to be similar to knee OCD, demonstrating the fibrosclerotic margins and possible articular cartilage fissuring or delamination (**Fig. 1**).[8,11]

The principles of treatment of the humeral OCD appear to be similar to that of knee OCD, at least based on the success reported in these few case reports at alleviating symptoms. The fact that some patients were treated conservatively, with good symptom resolution, must be tempered by the fact that the shoulder is not a weight-bearing joint. Therefore, even though some authors treated their patients conservatively with good symptom resolution, most recommend drilling of the sclerotic margin and intra-articular debridement of any cartilaginous injury, which includes both stable and unstable lesions, to heal the lesion.[7,9] The authors present 1 case of a 17-year-old patient who reported shoulder pain following several years of professional work pulling scallops up from the bottom of boxes in a rapid, repetitive fashion (see **Fig. 1**). After obtaining initial imaging (see **Fig. 1**A, B), he had a subsequent, unreported fall on the shoulder (disclosed to the surgeon postoperatively), 2 months after which, the rounded, chronic-appearing sclerotic loose body that was likely an in situ OCD was discovered and removed during arthroscopy. In order to prevent an engaging humeral defect, open treatment to debride the bony, avascular bed of the cystic tissue and fill the defect with iliac crest autograft with a fibrin glue sealant (see **Fig. 1**C) was performed. It is hoped that this may be his definitive treatment or a temporizing procedure prior to future resurfacing with autologous chondrocyte implantation or osteochondral allograft similar to a report in the literature.[10] His outcome is still pending at the time of this writing.

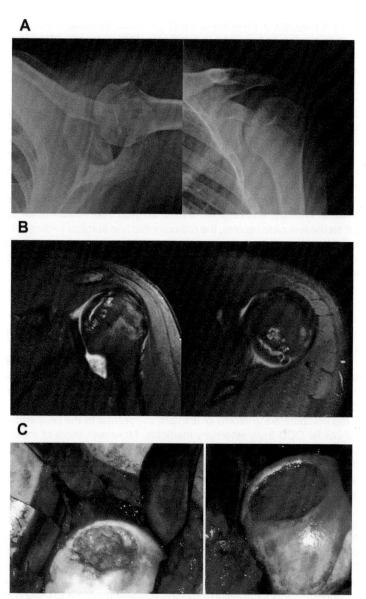

Fig. 1. Humeral head OCD in a 17-year-old scalloper with imaging 3 months prior to surgical intervention, with a significant interim fall on the arm. (*A*) Axillary and anterior-posterior radiographs at initial presentation. (*B*) MRI left shoulder T2 coronal fat saturation (FS) and proton density FS axial views demonstrating lesion instability. (*C*) Clinical photographs demonstrating appearance of humeral head at time of surgery and the appearance after bone grafting.

There are at least 10 cases reported of glenoid fossa OCD lesions in the literature, but with fewer publications overall.[15–20] The first report was in 1947, and it was presented with many other types of OCD.[18] It was not until 1990 that 2 case series were reported.[19,20] Similar to the humeral OCD variety, the glenoid fossa OCD is believed to be secondary to microtrauma at the shoulder,[15,20] and there is some evidence that it may occur predominately in overhead throwing athletes.[17,19] Once again, the radiographic appearance is similar to other anatomic sites, with radiolucency and sclerotic rims being the hallmark (**Fig. 2**A).[20]

Reported treatment of a glenoid fossa OCD has differed from humeral head OCDs, as the former appears to present most commonly with delamination or other injury to the articular cartilage. Surgical intervention is predominately debridement and removal of loose bodies,[16,19,20] but microfracture can be performed to stimulate articular fibrocartilaginous development.[16] The authors have utilized a trapdoor technique on a 15-year-old softball player that allows for debridement of fibrous tissue under the OCD with repair of a torn labrum, utilizing both suture anchors and the labral repair to secure the OCD into place, with good anecdotal results given the patient's current competitive play at the college level (see **Fig. 2**B, C).

Both humeral head and glenoid fossa OCDs appear to be rare, have a repetitive, microtraumautic etiology, and respond well to surgical intervention when symptomatic. Based on the few case reports, the radiographic and surgical findings of shoulder OCD suggest that these lesions can be ascribed to the same pathogenesis as OCD in other joints, at least as it relates to the provided definition of focal, subchondral bone involvement with risk of articular cartilage damage.

HIP OCD

At this time, the authors are unaware of an epidemiologic study attempting to determine the prevalence of hip OCD, specifically. Intuitively, it would seem that hip OCDs must occur with greater frequency than OCDs of the shoulder; except, close examination of the literature finds significant overlap between OCD and focal osteonecrosis of various etiologies. A search of PubMed using the keywords "osteochondritis dissecans hip" yielded 113 different publications in all languages. Few of these related to the comparative anatomy of animals, in contrast to the proliferative observation of shoulder OCD from veterinary medicine. Moreover, most of these publications would not qualify as OCD by the definition provided earlier in this article. Many reports discussed focal lesions with subchondral bone collapse, development of epiphyseal distortion with coxa magna, and subsequent articular loose body formation; these cases did not represent idiopathic presentations of these lesions.[21–25]

One of the primary overlapping pathologies reported in the literature is Legg-Calve-Perthes (LCP) disease.[21,22,25] There seems to be both a trend to identify LCP disease as an etiology for the femoral head OCD, and also to report both in the same article as if they represent similar pathologies.[22,25,26] Rowe and colleagues[22] suggested that 2% to 4% of LCP disease patients can develop OCD of the femoral head. Although this type of osteochondral lesion does not likely represent OCD in a pure form, it is important to recognize that this focal lesion may have a similar outcome to OCD in that it has a risk for developing loose bodies. When diagnosed, these authors suggest that surgical intervention is warranted with debridement of the hip joint.[21,22,25]

Besides LCP disease, there are a few other associated pathologies that may develop OCD of the femoral head; although, as with LCP, these may not be pure OCD lesions by definition. One example is a case series of an apparent familial form of femoral head OCD, but it is also associated with short stature and premature physeal closure with epiphyseal dysplasia.[24] There is also a report of association with developmental dysplasia of the hip.[21] Other reports are not as clear regarding the presence of a true OCD. One such report is of a middle-aged patient treated with an end-stage OCD lesion that presented purely as a loose body of unclear etiology.[27]

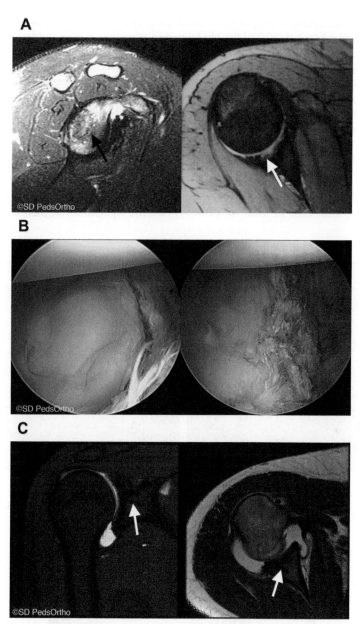

Fig. 2. OCD of the glenoid fossa in a 15-year-old softball player with concomitant posterior labral tear. (*A*) Initial presenting MRI, sagittal T2 FS and axial T1 demonstrating the lesion (*arrows*). (*B*) Arthroscopic photographs, initial view of glenoid surface and repeat arthroscopy 16 months later for recurrent internal impingement issues. (*C*) 16 months follow-up MRI, coronal T2 FS and axial T1 (*arrows* demonstrate suture anchors for repair of labrum and OCD). (*Courtesy of* SD PedsOrtho; with permission.)

Despite these confounding reports, there do appear to be a few case reports that may actually represent OCD of the hip joint, and they involve both the femoral head and the acetabulum.[23,25,26,28–32] Acetabulum OCD appears to be the rarest form of this pathology, occurring truly as singular case reports at least 3 times.[28,31,32] Each was confirmed by advanced imaging demonstrating findings most consistent with an OCD, and the treatment for each person was distinct, ranging from expectant observation to surgical dislocation and curettage of the lesion.[28,31] All 3 patients had symptoms at the hip that led them to be evaluated by an orthopedic surgeon. We present a fourth case report, courtesy of Dr Carl Nissen, of a skeletally immature patient with open triradiate cartilage and an acetabular OCD. **Figure 3**A demonstrates the pre-operative coronal MRI with unstable OCD sitting in situ. Moreover, **Figure 3**B is the sagittal MRI highlighting the location of the OCD relative to the triradiate cartilage. This patient was treated with arthroscopic removal of loose body that has, at least temporarily, relieved symptoms of pain at the hip (**Fig. 3**C).

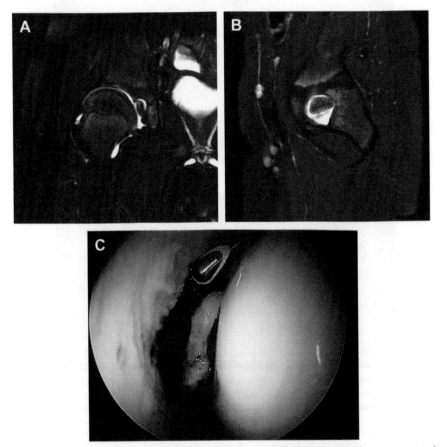

Fig. 3. A skeletally immature patient who presented with hip pain secondary to an acetabular OCD. (*A*) Initial presenting coronal T2 fat saturation MRI with unstable OCD sitting in situ. (*B*) Initial sagittal MRI, with the OCD apparently involving a portion of the open triradiate cartilage. (*C*) Intra-operative arthroscopic photograph, prior to insufflation with fluid, demonstrating the unstable acetabular OCD.

Femoral head OCD appears to be more common than that of the acetabulum,[23,25,26,29,30] although, due to the overlap and associated diagnosis of LCP in the literature, the true incidence is unknown.[23,25,26,29] Limiting the diagnosis of OCD of the femoral head to those cases when the rest of the femoral head appears normal,

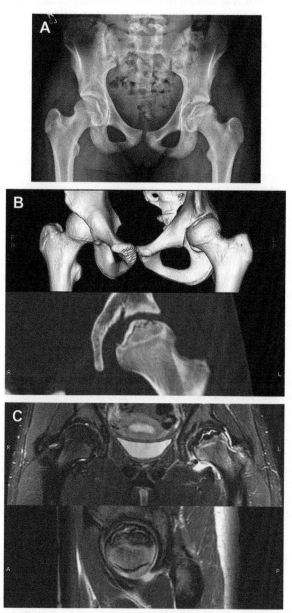

Fig. 4. Femoral head OCD in a 16-year-old Olympic hopeful gymnast with progressive hip pain. (*A*) Plain AP radiograph of her pelvis with OCD seen on left hip. (*B*) 3-dimemsional reconstruction and coronal CT scan image demonstrating size and location on the femoral head. (*C*) MRI coronal short T1 inversion recovery (STIR) and sagittal PD images demonstrating instability, as well as similarities to Perthes disease and other forms of avascular necrosis.

there are only 9 confirmed cases in the literature. It is possible however, that true end-stage OCDs of the femoral head are the normal sequelae of LCP disease. This is not clear in the literature.

Given that the differential diagnosis of these femoral head lesions is broader than that seen in other joints, it is difficult to identify specific clinical presentations, examination findings, or radiographic findings specific to femoral head OCD. It does seem clear, however, that patients can present in their youth or in adulthood, without gender predilection, and often with pain or limitations in hip motion (particularly in rotation).[23,25,30] These lesions are usually found by plain film (meaning that advanced imaging is not needed to identify the OCD) and by the fact that they are usually found adjacent to the fovea (**Fig. 4**A).[21] However, advanced imaging such as computed tomography (CT) or MRI can be important for treatment development and preoperative planning, such as in the 16-year-old gymnast who presented with hip pain, as shown in **Fig. 4**B, C. In evaluating these advanced images, the authors have noted that the femoral head OCD can cover a large area and is a source of confusion regarding the existence of focal OCD of the femoral head versus LCP disease and other forms of avascular necrosis.

The only consensus that can be pulled from the literature on femoral OCD is that surgery is often necessary to alleviate the patient's symptoms. Treatment includes debridement, removal of loose bodies, chondroplasty, and/or internal fixation of the lesion either performed with open arthrotomy or arthroscopy.[23,25,29,30] These same authors also discuss more significant surgeries in the form of osteotomy to alter the hip mechanics, but these appear to be performed primarily for the associated pathology found at the time of diagnosis. However, they mostly note resolution of the OCD with these procedures. For 1 case report of a lesion that was ultimately denuded of its articular cartilage, the authors report successful allograft resurfacing of the cartilage.[33]

SUMMARY

Being distinctly uncommon, the natural history, etiology, prognosis, and management of both shoulder and hip OCD are not known and not well studied. The various case reports in the literature suggest a few potential answers to this disease process, but by no means do they provide definitive recommendations. It appears that shoulder OCD, whether on the humeral head or the glenoid fossa, has relatively lower morbidity to the patient, possibly stemming from the fact that it is a nonweight-bearing joint. In contrast, it appears that many people with an OCD involving either the femoral head or the acetabulum may be destined to undergo surgery to alleviate their symptoms. Outcomes of hip OCD are clearly confounded by its association with other diseases, with notoriously poor outcomes and the significant concomitant procedures undertaken to address them.

The only recommendation that can be provided based on a review of the literature is to treat each patient individually, without specific evidence-based medicine outcomes to support care of the OCD lesion. It may be best to follow the research and outcomes of the capitellum OCD when making decisions regarding the care of shoulder OCD lesions, since these are both upper extremity, nonweight-bearing articulations. Furthermore, the treatment of hip OCD lesions may be best guided by the research done on knee OCD, because they share the similarity of a lower extremity, weight-bearing joint. Future research on these 2 uncommon varieties of OCD is critical and will require multicenter registries to enroll enough patients to help develop answers for natural history, outcomes, prognosis, and management.

REFERENCES

1. Edmonds EW, Polousky J. A review of knowledge in osteochondritis dissecans: 123 years of minimal evolution from Konig to the ROCK study group. Clin Orthop Relat Res 2013;471(4):1118–26.
2. Konig F. The classic: on loose bodies in the joint. 1887. Clin Orthop Relat Res 2013;471(4):1107–15.
3. Edmonds EW, Shea KG. Osteochondritis dissecans: editorial comment. Clin Orthop Relat Res 2013;471(4):1105–6.
4. Olstad K, Hendrickson EH, Carlson CS, et al. Transection of vessels in epiphyseal cartilage canals leads to osteochondrosis and osteochondrosis dissecans in the femoro-patellar joint of foals; a potential model of juvenile osteochondritis dissecans. Osteoarthr Cartil 2013;21(5):730–8.
5. Ytrehus B, Carlson CS, Ekman S. Etiology and pathogenesis of osteochondrosis. Vet Pathol 2007;44(4):429–48.
6. Kessler JI, Nikizad H, Shea KG, et al. The demographics and epidemiology of osteochondritis dissecans of the ankle, elbow, foot, and shoulder in children. Presented at the Annual Meeting of American Orthopedic Society of Sports Medicine. Chicago (IL), July 2013.
7. Anderson WJ, Guilford WB. Osteochondritis dissecans of the humeral head. An unusual cause of shoulder pain. Clin Orthop Relat Res 1983;(173):166–8.
8. Ganter M, Reichelt A. Osteochondrosis dissecans of the humeral head. Z Orthop Ihre Grenzgeb 1996;134(1):73–5 [in German].
9. Hamada S, Hamada M, Nishiue S, et al. Osteochondritis dissecans of the humeral head. Arthroscopy 1992;8(1):132–7.
10. Johnson DL, Warner JJ. Osteochondritis dissecans of the humeral head: treatment with a matched osteochondral allograft. J Shoulder Elbow Surg 1997; 6(2):160–3.
11. Lunden JB, Legrand AB. Osteochondritis dissecans of the humeral head. J Orthop Sports Phys Ther 2012;42(10):886.
12. Mahirogullari M, Chloros GD, Wiesler ER, et al. Osteochondritis dissecans of the humeral head. Joint Bone Spine 2008;75(2):226–8.
13. Miller LF, Hilkevitch A. Osteochondritis dissecans of the shoulder. Am J Roentgenol Radium Ther 1950;63(2):223–7 illust.
14. Pydisetty RV, Prasad SS, Kaye JC. Osteochondritis dissecans of the humeral head in an amateur boxer. J Shoulder Elbow Surg 2002;11(6):630–2.
15. Chu PJ, Shih JT, Hou YT, et al. Osteochondritis dissecans of the glenoid: a rare injury secondary to repetitive microtrauma. J Trauma 2009;67(3):E62–4.
16. Gogus A, Ozturk C. Osteochondritis dissecans of the glenoid cavity: a case report. Arch Orthop Trauma Surg 2008;128(5):457–60.
17. Koike Y, Komatsuda T, Sato K. Osteochondritis dissecans of the glenoid associated with the nontraumatic, painful throwing shoulder in a professional baseball player: a case report. J Shoulder Elbow Surg 2008;17(5):e9–12.
18. Lavner G. Osteochondritis dissecans; an analysis of forty-two cases and a review of the literature. Am J Roentgenol Radium Ther 1947;57(1):56–70.
19. Rossi F, Dragoni S. Osteochondrosis dissecans of the shoulder glenoid fossa diagnosed in four throwing athletes. J Sports Med Phys Fitness 2006;46(1):111–5.
20. Shanley DJ, Mulligan ME. Osteochondrosis dissecans of the glenoid. Skeletal Radiol 1990;19(6):419–21.
21. Linden B, Jonsson K, Redlund-Johnell I. Osteochondritis dissecans of the hip. Acta Radiol 2003;44(1):67–71.

22. Rowe SM, Chung JY, Moon ES, et al. Computed tomographic findings of osteo-chondritis dissecans following Legg-Calve-Perthes disease. J Pediatr Orthop 2003;23(3):356–62.

23. Siebenrock KA, Powell JN, Ganz R. Osteochondritis dissecans of the femoral head. Hip Int 2010;20(4):489–96.

24. Stattin EL, Tegner Y, Domellöf M, et al. Familial osteochondritis dissecans associated with early osteoarthritis and disproportionate short stature. Osteoarthr Cartil 2008;16(8):890–6.

25. Wood JB, Klassen RA, Peterson HA. Osteochondritis dissecans of the femoral head in children and adolescents: a report of 17 cases. J Pediatr Orthop 1995; 15(3):313–6.

26. Guilleminet M, Barbier JM. Osteochondritis dissecans of the hip. J Bone Joint Surg Br 1957;39(2):268–77 [in German].

27. Hagemann L, Berger S, Philipps B, et al. Osteochondrosis dissecans of the hip in adults—differential diagnosis of free joint bodies—case report. Z Orthop Ihre Grenzgeb 2006;144(3):301–4 [in German].

28. Hardy P, Hinojosa JF, Coudane H, et al. Osteochondritis dissecans of the acetabulum. Apropos of a case. Rev Chir Orthop Reparatrice Appar Mot 1992;78(2): 134–7 [in French].

29. Kerschbaumer F, Hausbrandt D, Bauer R. Long-term observation of osteo-chondrosis dissecans of the hip. Z Orthop Ihre Grenzgeb 1980;118(5):708–12 [in German].

30. Matsuda DK, Safran MR. Arthroscopic internal fixation of osteochondritis disse-cans of the femoral head. Orthopedics 2013;36(5):e683–6.

31. Werther K, Jensen KH. Osteochondritis dissecans of the acetabulum. Ugeskr Laeger 1997;159(22):3417–8.

32. Yildirim OS, Okur A, Erman Z. Osteochondritis dissecans of the acetabulum: a case report. Joint Bone Spine 2004;71(2):160–1.

33. Evans KN, Providence BC. Case report: fresh-stored osteochondral allograft for treatment of osteochondritis dissecans the femoral head. Clin Orthop Relat Res 2010;468(2):613–8.

Nonoperative Treatment of Osteochondritis Dissecans of the Knee

Justin S. Yang, MD, Ljiljana Bogunovic, MD, Rick W. Wright, MD*

KEYWORDS

- Osteochondritis dissecans • Juvenile osteochondritis dissecans
- Nonoperative treatment • Open physis • Stable lesions • Activity modification
- Return to play

KEY POINTS

- Osteochondritis dissecans is potentially devastating cause of knee pain in adolescents and adults.
- Prognosis and treatment is dependent on the stability of the lesion and the age of the patient. Skeletally immature patients with stable lesions are amenable for nonoperative treatment.
- Nonoperative treatment is less predictable in skeletally mature patients and patients with unstable lesions.
- Lesion size, location, and stability, along with symptomatology, should all be considered before initiating treatment.
- Modalities of nonoperative treatment can range from activity modification to complete immobilization. Close follow-up is recommended to monitor healing progression and symptom resolution.

INTRODUCTION

Osteochondritis dissecans (OCD) is an infrequent but potentially devastating cause of knee pain in adolescents and adults. First described by Paget in 1870, OCD involves a focal, idiopathic alteration of subchondral bone with risk for instability and disruption of adjacent articular cartilage that may result in premature arthritis.[1] Prognosis and treatment is dependent primarily on the stability of the lesion and the age of the patient. Although juvenile OCD generally presents as a stable lesion amenable to

Disclosures: The authors have no relevant disclosures to this article.
Department of Orthopedics, Washington University, 660 South Euclid MS 8233, St Louis, MO, USA
* Corresponding author.
E-mail address: wright@wudosis.wustl.edu

Clin Sports Med 33 (2014) 295–304
http://dx.doi.org/10.1016/j.csm.2013.11.003
0278-5919/14/$ – see front matter © 2014 Elsevier Inc. All rights reserved.

conservative treatment, symptomatic adult OCD lesions have diminished healing potential, are frequently unstable, and often require operative intervention. Numerous publications regarding the etiology, natural history, and treatment of OCD have been put forth; however, a general consensus remains elusive.

ETIOLOGY

The subchondral bone is the primary site of pathology in OCD lesions. The term osteochondritis dissecans, coined by Konig in 1888, is now recognized as a misnomer, as no evidence of an inflammatory process has ever been demonstrated in these lesions. Necrosis in the subchondral bone is a frequent but inconsistent histologic finding and the overlying articular cartilage is often normal.[2,3] Absent in the literature is a consensus as to whether subchondral bone necrosis is primary or secondary to the progression of OCD. These issues remain extremely relevant to the successful management options reviewed here.

The cause of OCD remains unknown, with several etiologies, including genetic predisposition, defective skeletal development, vascular insult, and trauma proposed in the literature. Usually no single causative factor can be identified and the true etiology is likely multifactorial. In discussing OCD lesions, one must be cautious to differentiate between the idiopathic type (topic of this review) and lesions resulting from osteonecrosis secondary to other factors, such as hemoglobinopathies, steroid use, and chemotherapy.

Familial inheritance has been suggested in several small studies involving multiple family members with OCD lesions.[4] In many of these familial cases, an association between dwarfism and short stature has been reported.[4–6] A sporadic form also has been identified, with no evidence of genetic predisposition or association with short stature.[7]

Ischemia was traditionally believed to be the primary cause of OCD lesions.[1] Issues such as emboli from blood or fat and/or disorders in subchondral vascular anatomy were felt to result in relative ischemia of the subchondral bone and subsequent subchondral fracture with fragment formation.[1,8] Trauma, specifically repetitive trauma, is currently the most accepted causative factor of OCD lesions. The association between OCD lesions and patient activity level supports this theory. In a study of more than 105 patients with OCD lesions involving the knee, 60% reported high-level participation in athletic activity.[9,10] The prevalence of OCD lesions has been shown to coincide with increased sports participation.[10] Repetitive trauma is believed to induce a stress reaction and subsequent stress fracture within the subchondral bone. In the setting of continued trauma or impaired healing capacity, fractured subchondral bone undergoes necrosis, leading to separation between the bone and overlying articular cartilage.

Altered joint mechanics also have been proposed as a factor contributing to the development of OCD lesions.[1,11] Lesions of the medial femoral condyle have been associated with varus alignment of the knee, whereas lesions of the lateral femoral condyle are more often seen in patients with valgus alignment.[12] The development of OCD lesions in the lateral femoral condyle also has been reported following saucerization of a discoid lateral meniscus.[13]

EPIDEMIOLOGY

The incidence of OCD is approximately 15 to 29 per 100,000 patients.[10,14] A steady rise in this number is likely secondary to increased provider awareness, more frequent use of advanced imaging, such as magnetic resonance imaging (MRI), introduction of sports at a younger age, increased intensity of sports participation, and early sport specialization. In general males are affected more often than females, with a reported male-to-female ratio of 5:3.[15] However, the gender gap is decreasing coincident with increased female sports participation. The age of presentation averages 14 years for juvenile lesions and 26 years for adult lesions.[16] Modern changes in sports participation also have impacted the age of presentation, with juvenile patients presenting at an increasingly younger age.[15]

PATIENT PRESENTATION

Most patients with OCD lesions present with vague complaints of knee pain and without a history of trauma.[1,11,17] The pain is generally nonspecific and difficult to localize, but is often activity related. Bent-knee activities, such as stair climbing, hill running, and prolonged sitting, tend to exacerbate symptoms. Adolescent and adult patients with unstable lesions may complain of mechanical symptoms of catching and locking and knee swelling.

PHYSICAL EXAMINATION

A thorough physical examination should be performed. Gait should be assessed for evidence of a limp. Patients with lesions involving the medial femoral condyle may ambulate with the affected limb held in external rotation. An effusion is present in approximately 20% of patients and is concerning for an unstable lesion.[18] The hip should be examined for evidence of pathology that could be contributing to referred knee pain. Quadriceps atrophy, if present, can be indicative of prolonged duration of symptoms. Crepitus with knee range of motion can occur with unstable lesions or a frank loose body. Tenderness is infrequently elicited over the antero-medial femoral condyle; the most common site of OCD lesions. The Wilson sign has been described as being specific to OCD lesions of the medial femoral condyle.[19] The test is performed with the knee flexed to 90° and the tibia externally rotated. The knee is than gradually extended. A positive test is when the patient experiences anteromedial pain as the knee approaches 30° of flexion and resolution of pain with internal tibial rotation. The Wilson maneuver is intended to produce impingement of the lateral aspect of the medial femoral condyle on the tibial spine, resulting in pain in the presence of a medial femoral condyle OCD lesion. The sensitivity of this test has been questioned, with a recent study reporting a negative result in 75% of patients with a radiographically evident OCD lesion, although resolution of a positive Wilson test has been associated with healing of the lesion.[20]

PROGNOSIS AND NATURAL HISTORY

The prognosis of OCD depends on the skeletal maturity of the patient and the stability of the lesion. Juvenile OCD occurs in patients with an open distal femoral physis and is associated with an increased healing capacity.[21] Stable OCD lesions are those with intact articular cartilage and a firm subchondral bone. In unstable lesions, there is often a break in the overlying cartilage with separation between the progeny and native bone and fragment formation. The fragment may reside within its bed (in situ) or may be completely detached as a loose body. These unstable lesions, especially in adults, follow a predictable progressive course of joint degeneration. Adolescents with closing physes pose a clinical challenge, as the healing potential in these patients is often difficult to predict.[21] The relationship between juvenile and adult OCD is not entirely understood. Although most adult lesions are believed to be juvenile lesions that have persisted, adult-onset lesions also have been described.[15]

IMAGING

Plain radiographs should be obtained in all patients with suspected OCD. The standard radiographic series includes weight-bearing anteroposterior, lateral view, the notch view to identify lesions on the posterior condyles, and a merchant view to assess the patellofemoral joint.[22] Plain radiographs are helpful in evaluating skeletal maturity, ruling out other bony injury, and determining the location and age of the lesion. Most lesions occur on the lateral aspect of the medial femoral condyle, but can be found in the lateral femoral condyle and patellofemoral joint. The radiographic appearance of the lesion changes with time. Early in the disease, a small radiolucency appears near the articular surface. As the lesions progress, a well-demarcated fragment may become visible with a clear demarcation of the progeny fragment from the native subchondral bone. Increased density of the fragment and sclerosis in the parent bed has been associated with increased chronicity of the lesion.[23] Plain radiographs in children younger than 7 should be viewed with caution. Normal anatomic variations in the distal femoral ossification center can be misinterpreted as OCD lesions.[24]

Advanced Imaging: Bone Scintigraphy and MRI

The ideal imaging modality will allow one to predict the stability and therefore healing potential of an OCD lesion. Despite the utility of plain radiographs, they are unreliable in assessing OCD lesion stability. Therefore, advanced imaging with bone scintigraphy and/or MRI has been used. Bone scintigraphy was first described by Cahill[15] as a method to assess lesion stability and monitor healing. Although this imaging modality was found to be reasonably reliable, the time-intensive nature of the technique, need for intravenous contrast, radiation exposure, and increased availability of MRI has resulted in less frequent use.

MRI has emerged as the gold standard in advanced imaging and is often used in the assessment of OCD lesions. Imaging with MRI allows for an estimation of lesion size and location and the status of the articular cartilage allowing for a prediction of lesion stability as well as other structures within the knee.[15,25,26] Several classification systems correlating MRI findings with arthroscopic grading of instability have been described. De Smet and colleagues[27] identified 4 MRI findings associated with lesion instability: (1) a high signal line (>5 mm) on T2 between the fragment and the subchondral bone, (2) homogeneous signal (>5 mm) below the lesion, (3) a break in the articular cartilage overlying the lesion, and (4) a high signal line extending from subchondral plate to the lesion. A high signal line on T2 sequence consistent with separation of the fragment and underlying bone was felt to be the best indicator of instability and is incorporated in the MRI OCD classification system described by Dipaola and colleagues.[27,28] Although highly sensitive, this MRI finding has been found to have low specificity, especially in skeletally immature patients.[16,29,30] O'Connor and colleagues[31] improved the accuracy of MRI in predicting stability of OCD lesions from 45% to 85% by classifying only those lesions with both a high signal line on T2 behind the fragment and a break in the articular cartilage on T1 as being unstable. Although MRI has emerged as the imaging technique of choice, there are no studies that have produced a valid and reliable set of criteria for using MRI as a prognosticator of care and outcomes.

NONOPERATIVE TREATMENT
Indications

The decision to treat an osteochondritis (OCD) lesion nonoperatively depends on the healing potential of the patient and of the lesion. Given the improved healing capacity of juvenile OCD, a trial of nonoperative treatment is attempted in most skeletally immature patients with stable lesions.[10,32,33] Characteristics commonly associated with failure of nonoperative treatment include skeletal maturity, large lesion size, abnormal location, instability, and mechanical symptomatology.[25,27,34–36] Healing potential decreases significantly with physeal closure, thus limiting the effectiveness of nonoperative treatment.[21] Larger lesions (>160–200 mm^2) have been associated with lower healing rates with nonoperative treatment.[27,34] Lesion instability, characterized by fluid signal behind the lesion on MRI, with articular cartilage breach and completely detached lesions are also a relative contraindication for conservative treatment.[14,27,35–37] Lesions in atypical locations, such as the non–weight-bearing portion of the lateral femoral condyle, are more likely to be unstable.[25] Mechanical symptoms, such as catching and locking, have been found to be an indicator of instability and an independent risk factor for failure.[34]

Nonoperative Regimens

Although many studies exist that compare nonoperative and surgical treatments for OCD lesions, there have been no studies directly comparing different regimens of nonoperative treatment. Indeed there is no consensus in the literature on what actually defines a nonoperative regimen. In most series, nonoperative management of OCD lesions consists of 3 main components: medication, activity modification, and immobilization.

Medication

There is only anecdotal evidence on the use of medication for symptom relief in OCD.[14,15,38] The 2 main medications used have been nonsteroidal anti-inflammatories (NSAIDs) and acetaminophen. Theoretical negative influences of NSAIDs on bone healing have led some investigators to recommend acetaminophen over NSAIDs.[38] In the end, both NSAIDs and acetaminophen, when prescribed, treat symptoms and seemingly have no affect on the outcome of OCD lesions.

Activity modification

In most series, the degree of activity modification depends predominantly on the patient's symptoms. If patients are symptomatic from sports-related activities, such as running or jumping, most investigators advocate the patients refrain from those activities. However, if the patient continues to be symptomatic with activities of daily living, such as walking, then progressive weight-bearing restrictions are used until the patient becomes asymptomatic.

Some modern protocols still advocate for immediate non–weight-bearing along with immobilization at initial presentation for a short duration of less than 6 weeks.[34] This should be considered in younger patients in whom compliance to activity modification and weight-bearing restrictions are an issue.

Immobilization

Historically, aggressive conservative treatments have used a long-leg cast and non–weight-bearing for periods of up to 18 months.[15] These protocols were shown to cause severe quadriceps atrophy, arthrofibrosis, and potential cartilage degeneration.[14,15] In modern protocols, immobilization of the knee can be prescribed either initially, or in a setting of continued pain with non–weight-bearing activity modification. Smillie[23] has suggested that immobilization should not exceed 4 months. A long-leg cast in slight flexion, a hinged brace, or knee immobilizer have all been used without comparisons among them. A long-leg cast offers rigid immobilization without issues of compliance. However, families often find them difficult, especially with showers and school. Knee immobilizers are easier to use for patients and family; however, knee stiffness and compliance can be an issue. Hinged knee and unloader braces can be used to allow limited motion at the knee while unloading pressure from the lesion. However, issues with pressure on the skin and tolerance in younger children limit their utility.[22] The American Academy of Orthopaedic Surgeons clinical practice guideline was unable to specifically recommend any one particular nonoperative treatment option (eg, activity restriction alone, casting, bracing) over another.[39]

Duration of Nonoperative Treatment and the Role of Imaging

For skeletally immature patients, nonoperative treatment durations have been published ranging from 3 months to 2 years.[14,32,34–37,40] For stable lesions in skeletally immature patients, a minimum of 6 to 12 months of nonoperative treatment has been recommended before operative intervention.[34,37,40] During this time, progression of healing should be followed. Wall and colleagues[34] reported 66% of stable juvenile OCD lesions will show progressive healing in a 6-month period. Krause and colleagues[37] reported that 33% of the patients showed healing progression within 6 months, and an additional 24% of patients can show healing progression between 6 and 12 months. Cahill and colleagues[40] reported that 57% of stable juvenile OCD will heal within 10 to 18 months. We believe as long as progressive healing is seen, the nonoperative treatment should be continued. For patients nearing skeletal maturity, most investigators have recommended at least a 3-month nonoperative trial.[14,15,32] In skeletally mature patients with stable lesions, several investigators have recommended a minimum of 3 months of nonoperative treatment.[1,14]

Radiographic and clinical follow-up should occur at 6-week to 8-week intervals during nonoperative treatment.[34,37,40] Progression of healing on imaging and decrease in symptoms should be assessed at each follow-up. Early radiographic and MRI healing can be seen as early as 4 weeks in some series; however, complete radiographic healing and remodeling of OCD lesions can take up to 2 years.[21,27,33,37,40,41] On radiographic follow-up, progressive reossification of the lesion should be seen.[34] On MRI, healing or progression toward healing was defined as lesion size reduction by at least 15% and reduction of high signal around the lesion.[27,37] Although it is no longer commonly used, bone scintigraphy can play a role in assessing healing as well with interval scans every 4 months, with healing defined as less than stage II of activity.[11,40]

Return to Sports and Follow-up

After healing is seen on imaging, a slow gradual return to asymptomatic activities and sports should be instituted. As healing progresses, low-impact recreational activities, such as cycling, swimming, walking, and lower extremity strength training are added, provided the patient remains asymptomatic. Complete healing of the lesion should be seen on imaging before allowing the patient to return to high-impact activities and competitive sports.[15,33,34] For skeletally immature patients who have healed, some investigators advocate for 6 to 12 months of follow-up or until skeletal maturity to monitor the lesion.[15,36]

OUTCOMES OF NONOPERATIVE TREATMENT

The healing rates with nonoperative treatment have varied widely from 49% to 96% in published series. The variability in part is seen due to the mixture of skeletally immature and mature patients in most series.

The most successful study reported to date on nonoperative treatment of OCD lesions was done by Sales de Gauzy and colleagues.[33] They conducted a retrospective review of 31 juvenile OCD lesions in 24 patients younger than 11. The only treatment they received was discontinuation of sports activities. Thirty (96%) of the lesions healed on radiographs with nonoperative management.[33] Unfortunately, lesion size and duration of treatment were not reported.

Hughston and colleagues[14] reported on a mixed cohort of 15 juvenile OCD and 7 adult OCD lesions (18 patients) with a mean age of 16.7 years (range 8–44) treated nonoperatively. Three of the knees were asymptomatic at the time of presentation. The protocol used was activity restriction and quad exercises. Hughston and colleagues[14] noted that 82% of patients treated nonoperatively had good or excellent rating. They did note that the nonoperative group on average had smaller lesions than the surgical group.

Cahill and colleagues[40] prospectively followed 92 OCD lesions in 76 patients with an average age at presentation of 12.5 years. All patients were participants in athletics or exercise programs. All patients were conservatively treated with activity modification and weight-bearing restrictions if persistently symptomatic. No immobilization was used. Healing was followed using bone scintigraphy every 8 weeks. Forty lesions eventually failed to show progression of healing on scintigraphy and underwent surgery. The investigators concluded smaller lesion size showed a moderate correlation toward success. Stability of the lesion based on MRI was not examined.

More recent studies have been more focused in terms of patient population and lesion stability. Wall and colleagues[34] followed 47 radiographically stable juvenile OCD lesions (42 patients). Stability of the lesion was initially assessed with both radiographs and MRI. All patients were managed with 6 weeks of cast immobilization followed by knee unloader bracing and activity restriction for 6 months total. Serial radiographs were taken every 6 weeks for up to 6 months to determine healing progression. After 6 months of nonoperative management, 16 (34%) of the 47 lesions had failed to progress toward healing. Of the 31 lesions (66%) that were progressing toward healing, 7 had completely reossified at the time of the 6-month evaluation.

Another recent retrospective study reported on 76 stable juvenile OCD lesions in 62 patients. All patients were treated with activity modification and weight-bearing restrictions until they were pain free for 12 months. MRI scans were used on presentation to determine the stability of the lesion, and again at the 6-month and 12-month follow-up to determine healing progression. After 6 months of nonoperative treatment, 25 (33%) of 76 lesions had progressed toward healing. After 12 months, 37 lesions (49%) had progressed toward healing.

Long-term follow-up radiographs after successful treatment of OCDs in skeletally immature patients have not shown signs of early osteoarthritis.[10,33] However, skeletally mature patients with healed OCDs showed an onset of arthritis 10 years earlier than average.[10,33]

SUMMARY

The decision to treat OCD lesions nonoperatively should be based on the individual patient and his or her lesion healing potential. Lesion size, location, and stability, along with symptomatology, should all be considered. A trial of nonoperative treatment should be used initially in skeletally immature patients with stable lesions for a minimum of 3 months, with reported success rate ranging from 50% to 96%. Modalities of nonoperative treatment can range from activity modification to complete immobilization. Close follow-up is recommended to monitor healing progression and symptom resolution. Additional research is necessary to improve the predictive ability of nonoperative management, including correlating lesion size, stability, and healing, and comparing different nonoperative treatment approaches.

REFERENCES

1. Edmonds EW, Polousky J. A review of knowledge in osteochondritis dissecans: 123 years of minimal evolution from Konig to the ROCK study group. Clin Orthop Relat Res 2013;471(4):1118–26.
2. Yonetani Y, Nakamura N, Natsuume T, et al. Histological evaluation of juvenile osteochondritis dissecans of the knee: a case series. Knee Surg Sports Traumatol Arthrosc 2010;18(6):723–30.
3. Uozumi H, Sugita T, Aizawa T, et al. Histologic findings and possible causes of osteochondritis dissecans of the knee. Am J Sports Med 2009;37(10): 2003–8.
4. Mubarak SJ, Carroll NC. Familial osteochondritis dissecans of the knee. Clin Orthop Relat Res 1979;(140):131–6.
5. Andrew TA, Spivey J, Lindebaum RH. Familial osteochondritis dissecans and dwarfism. Acta Orthop Scand 1981;52(5):519–23.
6. Stattin E, Tegner Y, Domellof M, et al. Familial osteochondritis dissecans associated with early osteoarthritis and disproportionate short stature. Osteoarthritis Cartilage 2008;16(8):890–6.
7. Petrie PW. Aetiology of osteochondritis dissecans. Failure to establish a familial background. J Bone Joint Surg Br 1977;59(3):366–7.
8. Clanton TO, DeLee JC. Osteochondritis dissecans. History, pathophysiology and current treatment concepts. Clin Orthop Relat Res 1982;(167):50–64.
9. Aichroth P. Osteochondritis dissecans of the knee. A clinical survey. J Bone Joint Surg Br 1971;53(3):440–7.
10. Linden B. The incidence of osteochondritis dissecans in the condyles of the femur. Acta Orthop Scand 1976;47(6):664–7.
11. Kocher M, Tucker R, Ganley T, et al. Management of osteochondritis dissecans of the knee: current concepts review. Am J Sports Med 2006;34(7):1181–91.
12. Jacobi M, Wahl P, Bouaicha S, et al. Association between mechanical axis of the leg and osteochondritis dissecans of the knee: radiographic study on 103 knees. Am J Sports Med 2010;38(7):1425–8.
13. Hashimoto Y, Yoshida G, Tomihara T, et al. Bilateral osteochondritis dissecans of the lateral femoral condyle following bilateral total removal of lateral discoid meniscus: a case report. Arch Orthop Trauma Surg 2008;128(11):1265–8.
14. Hughston JC, Hergenroeder PT, Courtenay BG. Osteochondritis dissecans of the femoral condyles. J Bone Joint Surg Am 1984;66(9):1340–8.
15. Cahill BR. Osteochondritis dissecans of the knee: treatment of juvenile and adult forms. J Am Acad Orthop Surg 1995;3(4):237–47.
16. Kijowski R, Blankenbaker D, Shinki K, et al. Juvenile versus adult osteochondritis dissecans of the knee: appropriate MR imaging criteria for instability. Radiology 2008;248(2):571–8.
17. Glancy GL. Juvenile osteochondritis dissecans. Am J Knee Surg 1999;12(2): 120–4.

18. Hefti F, Bequiristain J, Krauspe R, et al. Osteochondritis dissecans: a multicenter study of the European Pediatric Orthopedic Society. J Pediatr Orthop B 1999; 8(4):231–45.
19. Wilson JN. A diagnostic sign in osteochondritis dissecans of the knee. J Bone Joint Surg Am 1967;49(3):477–80.
20. Conrad JM, Stanitski CL. Osteochondritis dissecans: Wilson's sign revisited. Am J Sports Med 2003;31(5):777–8.
21. Paletta F, Bednarz P, Stanitski C, et al. The prognostic value of quantitative bone scan in knee osteochondritis dissecans. A preliminary experience. Am J Sports Med 1998;26(1):7–14.
22. Schulz JF, Chambers HG. Juvenile osteochondritis dissecans of the knee: current concepts in diagnosis and management. Instr Course Lect 2013;62:455–67.
23. Smillie IS. Treatment of osteochondritis dissecans. J Bone Joint Surg Br 1957; 39(2):248–60.
24. Milgram JW. Radiological and pathological manifestations of osteochondritis dissecans of the distal femur. A study of 50 cases. Radiology 1978;126(2):305–11.
25. Samora W, Chevillet J, Adler B, et al. Juvenile osteochondritis dissecans of the knee: predictors of lesion stability. J Pediatr Orthop 2012;32(1):1–4.
26. Quatman C, Hettrich C, Schmitt L, et al. The clinical utility and diagnostic performance of MRI for identification and classification of knee osteochondritis dissecans. J Bone Joint Surg Am 2012;94(11):1036–44.
27. De Smet AA, Ilahi OA, Graf BK. Untreated osteochondritis dissecans of the femoral condyles: prediction of patient outcome using radiographic and MR findings. Skeletal Radiol 1997;26(8):463–7.
28. Dipaola JD, Nelson DW, Colville MR. Characterizing osteochondral lesions by magnetic resonance imaging. Arthroscopy 1991;7(1):101–4.
29. Heywood C, Benke M, Brindle K, et al. Correlation of magnetic resonance imaging to arthroscopic findings of stability in juvenile osteochondritis dissecans. Arthroscopy 2011;27(2):194–9.
30. Yoshida S, Ikata T, Takai H, et al. Osteochondritis dissecans of the femoral condyle in the growth stage. Clin Orthop Relat Res 1998;(346):162–70.
31. O'Connor M, Palaniappan M, Khan N, et al. Osteochondritis dissecans of the knee in children. A comparison of MRI and arthroscopic findings. J Bone Joint Surg Br 2002;84(2):258–62.
32. Lindholm TS, Osterman K. Treatment of juvenile osteochondritis dissecans in the knee. Acta Orthop Belg 1979;45(6):633–40.
33. Sales de Gauzy J, Mansat C, Darodes P, et al. Natural course of osteochondritis dissecans in children. J Pediatr Orthop B 1999;8(1):26–8.
34. Wall E, Vourazeris J, Myer G, et al. The healing potential of stable juvenile osteochondritis dissecans knee lesions. J Bone Joint Surg Am 2008;90(12):2655–64.
35. Pill S, Ganley T, Milam R, et al. Role of magnetic resonance imaging and clinical criteria in predicting successful non-operative treatment of osteochondritis dissecans in children. J Pediatr Orthop 2003;23(1):102–8.
36. Cepero S, Ullot R, Sastre S. Osteochondritis of the femoral condyles in children and adolescents: our experience over the last 28 years. J Pediatr Orthop B 2005;14(1):24–9.
37. Krause M, Hapfelmeier A, Moller M, et al. Healing predictors of stable juvenile osteochondritis dissecans knee lesions after 6 and 12 months of non-operative treatment. Am J Sports Med 2013;41(10):2384–91.
38. Crawford DC, Safran MR. Osteochondritis dissecans of the knee. J Am Acad Orthop Surg 2006;14(2):90–100.

39. Chambers HG, Shea KG, Carey JL. AAOS clinical practice guideline: diagnosis and treatment of osteochondritis dissecans. J Am Acad Orthop Surg 2011;19(5):307–9.
40. Cahill BR, Phillips MR, Navarro R. The results of conservative management of juvenile osteochondritis dissecans using joint scintigraphy. A prospective study. Am J Sports Med 1989;17(5):601–5 [discussion: 605–6].
41. Detterline A, Goldstein J, Rue J, et al. Evaluation and treatment of osteochondritis dissecans lesions of the knee. J Knee Surg 2008;21(2):106–15.

Drilling Techniques for Osteochondritis Dissecans

Benton E. Heyworth, MD[a],*, Eric W. Edmonds, MD[b,c],
M. Lucas Murnaghan, MD, MEd, FRCSC[d,e], Mininder S. Kocher, MD[a]

KEYWORDS

- Osteochondritis dissecans • Drilling • Knee

KEY POINTS

- Isolated drilling of an osteochondritis dissecans lesion (OCD), currently performed as an arthroscopic procedure, is most commonly indicated for stable lesions in skeletally immature patients for whom nonoperative treatments fail.
- Drilling is designed to disrupt the sclerotic margin of a nonhealing OCD lesion and introduce biologic factors from the adjacent healthy cancellous bone to stimulate healing.
- Three techniques of drilling are most commonly used in the knee, including (1) transarticular drilling, which involves drilling through the articular cartilage to reach the affected subchondral bone under arthroscopic visualization; (2) retroarticular drilling, in which fluoroscopic guidance of Kirschner wire (K-wire) placement allows sparing of the articular cartilage; and (3) notch drilling, wherein the K-wire is placed behind the involved articular surface via entry through the intercondylar notch.
- Based on multiple reports in the literature, all 3 techniques of drilling have demonstrated high rates of OCD healing and good return to function among studied populations. Because no single technique has demonstrated clear superiority, comparative studies are needed to better elucidate the relative advantages and disadvantages of the techniques.

INTRODUCTION

Osteochondritis dissecans (OCD) is an uncommon, idiopathic disease of subchondral bone, in which disrupted or decreased blood supply to a focal region of bone adjacent to the articular cartilage can lead to softening, fissuring, delamination, and/or frank separation of a segment of the articular surface.[1–3] Although OCD has been reported

[a] Division of Sports Medicine, Department of Orthopedic Surgery, Boston Children's Hospital, Harvard Medical School, 300 Longwood Avenue, Boston, MA 02115, USA; [b] Division of Orthopedic Surgery, Rady Children's Hospital, 3030 Children's Way, San Diego, CA 92123, USA; [c] Department of Orthopedic Surgery, University of California San Diego, 200 West Arbor Drive, CA 92103, USA; [d] Department of Surgery, University of Toronto, Toronto, Ontario, Canada; [e] Division of Orthopaedics, The Hospital for Sick Children, Toronto, Ontario, Canada
* Corresponding author. 300 Longwood Avenue, Hunnewell 217, Boston, MA 02115.
E-mail address: benton.heyworth@childrens.harvard.edu

Clin Sports Med 33 (2014) 305–312
http://dx.doi.org/10.1016/j.csm.2013.11.007
0278-5919/14/$ – see front matter © 2014 Elsevier Inc. All rights reserved.

to occur in a variety of joints, including the ankle, elbow, and, more rarely, the shoulder and hip, by far the most commonly affected joint is the knee, with disproportionate involvement of the femoral condyles. Therefore, this report focuses on the techniques used for the treatment of knee OCD. However, the principles of drilling may be generally applicable to all joints, with subtle management differences based on location.

Although OCD has been described in adult patients, it is chiefly considered to be a condition of childhood and adolescence, affecting the developing subchondral bone in the skeletally immature patient. Therefore, treatment of juvenile OCD (JOCD) has been the focus of most reports in the literature, with an emphasis on stimulating healing of the subchondral bone before the condition progresses to more advanced stages, for which more technically challenging and invasive techniques, such as fixation and articular resurfacing procedures, are required to prevent arthritis and disability. Stable JOCD lesions primarily involve changes to the subchondral bone without disruption of the smooth surface of overlying articular cartilage. These stable lesions are initially treated with nonoperative methods, such as activity modification (eg, restriction from sports or impact activities), crutch weight-bearing protection, unloader bracing, and brace or cast immobilization.[2,3] When these nonoperative modalities fail to heal the OCD (or incomplete healing occurs), then the gold standard for treatment is drilling of the lesion, in which a small K-wire is generally used to disrupt the sclerotic margin of a nonhealing OCD lesion. The theory of this surgical management is that the disruption of the sclerotic margin introduces biologic factors from the surrounding healthy cancellous bone to stimulate healing. This report describes 3 of the most common techniques of drilling, with an emphasis on the technical aspects and theoretical advantages or disadvantages of each.

TRANSARTICULAR DRILLING

The technique of transarticular drilling begins with arthroscopic assessment of the OCD lesion, which includes both direct visualization of the appearance of the lesion, and palpation of the margins of the lesion and the surrounding cartilage with an arthroscopic probe. If significant disruption of the contour of the articular cartilage is present, or if gross mobility of the lesion or significant chondral fissuring is seen, consideration of the addition of fixation of the lesion should be made, because occasionally progression of the lesion to an unstable status may have occurred between the time of the most recent MRI and surgery, or the MRI may have failed to reveal certain signs of instability seen during surgery. However, if the lesion is instead deemed to be stable, and the margins of the lesion are clearly delineated, usually through identification of softer cartilage at the transition between affected and unaffected underlying subchondral bone, attention is turned toward drilling of the lesion. Drilling is performed with a small K-wire, most commonly either a 0.062 or 0.045 inches, although the latter is currently favored by most surgeons to minimize disruption of the articular cartilage. The wire is used to penetrate the lesion precisely perpendicular to the chondral surface with a wire driver (**Fig. 1**A), which often requires introducing the wire percutaneously at several different sites, with varying degrees of flexion or extension of the knee to achieve perpendicularity. Care is taken to advance the wire an appropriate depth through the affected subchondral bone to the deeper, healthier cancellous bone (see **Fig. 1**B), after which fat bubbles or bleeding from the marrow may be seen intra-articularly (see **Fig. 1**C). Although overpenetration to the depth of the distal femoral physis should be avoided, no growth disturbances have been reported in association with this technique. The number of penetrations of the Kirschner wire (K-wire) depends on the size of the K-wire and the size of the lesion, although previous

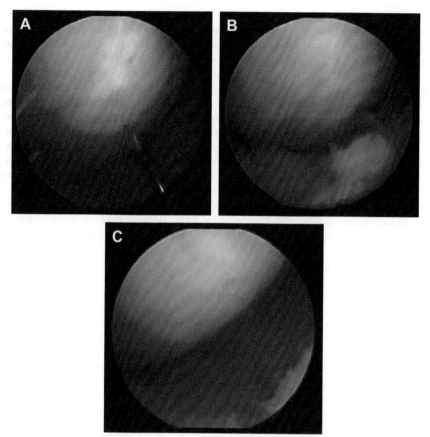

Fig. 1. (A) Arthroscopic photographs showing perpendicular K-wire placement during trans-articular drilling technique. (B) K-wire penetration of the OCD lesion. (C) Fat bubbles confirming adequate penetration of the healthy cancellous marrow of the femoral condyle, deep to the affected subchondral bone.

studies have referred to use of between 6 and 10 passes of the wire,[4] with the multiple passes attempting to uniformly cover the lesion,[5] being separated by several millimeters so as not to disrupt the macroarchitecture or stability of the lesion. Postoperatively, most authors institute a period of weight-bearing protection for 6 weeks, with initiation of formal physical therapy to facilitate early resumption of normal range of motion and, later, a weight-bearing strengthening program. Serial radiographs are obtained at follow-up visits every 6 to 12 weeks postoperatively to assess the bony healing of the lesion.

The primary advantage of the transarticular technique is its relative technical simplicity, the direct visualization of K-wire placement relative to the margins of the lesion, and optimization of the spacing and coverage of drilling passes. In addition, although the occasional stable OCD will demonstrate such smooth contour of the articular surface that fluoroscopic guidance is warranted to confirm the location of the lesion and drilling placement, most cases do not require radiographic assistance.

Several retrospective series have demonstrated the high rates of healing and low morbidity associated with the procedure. Aglietti and colleagues[6] described full healing by a mean of 4.9 months in 16 knees in 14 children with a mean age of 12.8 years.

At a mean of 4.7 years follow-up, all children remained asymptomatic, with all children having returned to their baseline activity level, including impact athletics. Anderson and colleagues[5] reported healing, return to sports, and "normal" or "near-normal" scores on the International Knee Documentation Committee (IKDC) questionnaire in 18 of 20 lesions (90%) by a mean of 4 months in skeletally immature knees. Because only 2 of 4 lesions (50%) in skeletally mature knees in the series healed, the authors recommended alternative primary treatment of stable OCD lesions in patients with closed physes. All 30 knees in 23 children with open physes described by Kocher and colleagues[4] demonstrated healing by a mean of 4.4 months (range, 1–11 months), with the mean Lysholm score improving from 58 to 93 and regression analysis correlating younger age with the degree of score improvement. Gunton and colleagues[7] recently investigated drilling techniques through a systematic review of the literature, and included 2 other studies on the transarticular approach, in addition to 3 studies described above. The authors pooled the results of the studies' subjects, concluding that transarticular drilling demonstrated a 91% healing rate at an average of 4.5 months. No complications were reported in any of the 5 studies included.

RETROARTICULAR DRILLING

Arthroscopic assessment of the OCD lesion before retroarticular drilling is performed in similar fashion to that described for transarticular drilling. After confirmation of lesion stability, the arthroscopy equipment is removed from the joint and a C-arm fluoroscopy unit is set up for an anteroposterior view of the knee (**Fig. 2**A). A 0.062- or 0.045-inch K-wire is placed percutaneously through the cortex of the affected condyle, just distal to the distal femoral physis, and advanced so that the tip of the wire penetrates the center of the most distal aspect of OCD lesion, without penetrating the articular surface (see **Fig. 2**B). With the K-wire left in place, the orientation of the fluoroscopic C-arm is then shifted to obtain a true lateral view of the femoral condyles, with the introduction of a second wire, if necessary, to achieve a perfect center-center position of the wire within the OCD lesion in both planes (see **Fig. 2**C). This guiding K-wire is then cut short outside of the skin to allow the unobstructed passage of additional K-wires for penetration around the initial wire. The additional passes are made under fluoroscopic guidance via rotation of a parallel wire guide circumferentially around the guiding K-wire in 1-mm increments and sufficient distance from the initial wire, so as to drill the entire OCD lesion, depending on its size. In one described technique,[8] the authors report the desired tactile sensation during wire advancement of encountering a "hard end point," representing the wire reaching the proximal margin of the lesion, with a subsequent "breakthrough sensation" signifying the disruption of the sclerotic rim and penetration of the wire into the most distal subchondral extent of lesion. Edmonds and colleagues[9] approximated 15 to 20 wire passes, each with a new percutaneous entry through the skin with the 0.062-inch K-wire, being optimal to achieve adequate drilling in their series, whereas Donaldson and Wojtys[10] recommended making a small skin incision over the condyle, through which to advance the K-wire, which they passed 4 to 8 times into the lesion. The postoperative rehabilitation and monitoring approaches after this technique are similar to those used after transarticular drilling.

The primary advantage of the retroarticular technique, compared with the transarticular technique, is the preservation of the articular cartilage. The intraepiphyseal approach may allow for more K-wire penetrations, and therefore greater disruption of the sclerotic margin of the OCD lesion without concern for chondral injury. This technique may also allow better access to far posterior condylar OCD lesions, for

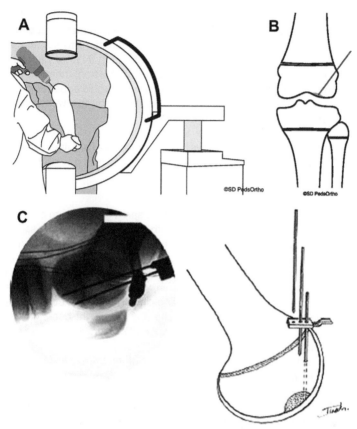

Fig. 2. (*A*) Intraoperative setup for retroarticular drilling. (*B*) Clinical photograph, antero-posterior fluoroscopic view, and schematic showing desired technique for retroarticular drilling. (*C*) Lateral fluoroscopic view (*left*) and schematic (*right*) showing desired technique for retroarticular drilling.

which perpendicular K-wire passage can be difficult to visualize intra-articularly with the transarticular approach. Disadvantages include a slightly more involved intraoperative setup, the need for optimal fluoroscopic visualization of the margins of the lesion in 2 planes, and the radiation exposure that stems from the required use of fluoroscopy.

Several level IV studies have emerged describing the results of retroarticular drilling, also referred to as *extra-articular drilling*. Donaldson and Wojtys[10] followed 12 of 15 skeletally immature patients who underwent drilling via the above technique for an average of 21 months (range, 8–38 months). In 12 knees, full radiographic healing, complete return to activities, and normal knee examinations were reported by 8.5 months postoperatively, whereas one patient's lesion progressed to instability and had a "fair" result in the follow-up period.

Edmonds and colleagues[9] reported a mean time to healing of 11.8 months (range, 1.3–47.3 months) and a mean time of return to activities of 2.8 months (range, 1.3–13.1 months) in 59 children with stable lesions who underwent retroarticular drilling. Importantly, the authors noted that large lesions (>320 mm^2) required a longer time to healing, averaging 15.3 months, compared with small lesions (<320 mm^2), which healed within an average of 8.3 months. Among patients in this series, 13% underwent subsequent procedures, such as repeat drilling, fixation, or bone grafting. Boughanem and colleagues[8] investigated the technique in 31 skeletally immature patients, finding significant improvement in Lysholm scores from a mean of 70 to 95, and scores on the visual analog scale for pain from 6.9 to 1.3. Although 94% of patients showed improvement in the radiographic appearance of the OCD lesion, mean time to healing was not reported, 2 patients showed no change in radiographic appearance, and 1 patient underwent 2 subsequent procedures within the study follow-up period, which averaged 4 years in the study population.

Gunton and colleagues[7] assessed a total of 6 studies on retroarticular drilling, including those by Donaldson and Wotjys[10] and Edmonds et al,[9] finding an 86% healing rate at 5.6 months, with no perioperative complications in any of the series.

NOTCH DRILLING

Drilling through the intercondylar notch follows the same general surgical principles as the 2 techniques described earlier, starting with an arthroscopic assessment of the OCD lesion. Kawasaki and colleagues[11] describe introducing a 1.5-mm K-wire through the anteromedial or anterolateral portal for drilling of a lateral or medial femoral condyle OCD lesion, respectively. The wire is advanced into the "bare area" of the intercondylar space, just behind the lesion, with "more than three K-wires" being inserted through the lesion into the healthy cancellous bone of the condyle (**Fig. 3**A). In contrast to previous reports, these authors allowed full weight-bearing 1 week after the procedure, with early active and passive range of motion, and the use of a continuous passive motion machine.

Notch drilling combines some of the advantages of the transarticular technique (eg, the vector of K-wire passing into the lesion can be visualized directly arthroscopically during the procedure without requiring fluoroscopy in most cases) with the primary advantage of the retroarticular technique (ie, penetration of the articular cartilage overlying the affected subchondral bone is avoided). The disadvantage of this technique is that the channels created by K-wire passage may not allow for penetration of significant portions of affected subchondral bone (see **Fig. 3**B), particularly with OCD lesions occurring in the center of the condyle. The technique may therefore have slightly more limited applicability than the other two described techniques, and may be best utilized only for those lesions directly adjacent to the notch, ie, the far lateral aspect of the

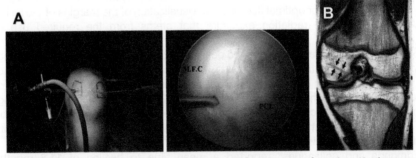

Fig. 3. (A) Intercondylar notch drilling. (B) MR image showing site of previous K-wire passage from intercondylar notch drilling (*arrows*) in a healing OCD lesion. (*From* [A] Kawasaki K, Uchioa Y, Adachi N, et al. Drilling from the intercondylar area for treatment of osteochondritis dissecans of the knee joint. Knee 2003;10(3):260, Fig. 2, with permission; and [B] Kawasaki K, Uchioa Y, Adachi N, et al. Drilling from the intercondylar area for treatment of osteochondritis dissecans of the knee joint. Knee 2003;10(3):262, Fig. 5, with permission.)

medial femoral condyle (a common location) and the far medial aspect of the lateral femoral condyle (an uncommon location).

Kawasaki and colleagues[11] reported radiographic healing after notch drilling of all 16 knees in 11 skeletally immature patients and 1 skeletally mature patient at a mean of 4 months postoperatively. MRI was also used to assess postsurgical healing, with a time to healing lagging behind radiographic healing by 3 months, at an average of 7 months. Mean Lysholm scores improved from a mean of 70.4 preoperatively to 97.8 postoperatively. No perioperative complications were reported and no revision surgeries were performed at a mean of 16 months (range, 12–24 months).

AUTHORS' PREFERRED TECHNIQUE

Both the transarticular and retroarticular techniques, as described earlier, are safe and effective, and are interchangeably used for OCD lesions in various locations of the knee. Transarticular drilling is often preferred, because it allows reliable visualization of entry of the K-wire directly into the lesion, with a desired coverage and spacing of drilling passes. For obviously stable lesions, which are seen clearly on plain radiographs but with margins that may not be clearly identifiable through arthroscopic assessment because of minimal tactile or visual cues on the chondral surface, retroarticular techniques may be preferable because of the reliance on fluoroscopic localization and the sparing of the articular cartilage overlying the lesion. In addition, retroarticular drilling is preferred for far-posterior condylar lesions, for which transarticular drilling may be difficult to perform because of the required hyperflexion of the knee, which pulls the capsule tightly against the condyle and makes arthroscopic visualization challenging. Notch drilling, although rarely performed in isolation, may be used in conjunction with either of the other two techniques for transarticular drilling for far-medial lesions of the lateral femoral condyle and the classic far-lateral lesions of the medial femoral condyle, as a means of ensuring disruption of the involved subchondral bone with relative sparing of the articular cartilage.

Postoperative rehabilitation protocols and return-to-sport criteria remain variable among authors and a subject of ongoing controversy.[2–4,8] The authors believe that weight-bearing protection with crutches for approximately 6 weeks after drilling provides the healing subchondral bone with the most favorable healing environment while minimizing the chances of lesion collapse or progression to instability. However, immediate non–weight-bearing range-of-motion exercises are used in conjunction with crutch protection to optimize cartilage metabolism after drilling. Return to sports is considered based on both radiographic progression of healing and a patient's signs and symptoms in the postoperative follow-up period. Significant or near-complete healing of the subchondral bone on radiographs or MRI should be seen before cutting, pivoting, and impact activities are allowed. Moreover, complete resolution of both pain and intra-articular effusion, and demonstration of symmetric quad and hamstring strength and dynamic knee stability, provides young patients with the greatest opportunity for successful return to athletics without risk of additional injury. Although persistence or recurrent progression of a healing, stable OCD lesion toward instability is a rarely seen phenomenon, the authors believe that radiographic and clinical monitoring of patients with OCD for at least 1 year after return to activities is also important to ensure the long-term health of the young athlete's knee.

SUMMARY

Drilling of OCD, when pursued for skeletally immature patients with stable OCD lesions that do not demonstrate healing with conservative measures, is highly effective at stimulating radiographic healing of the affected subchondral bone and allowing for a good return to function and sports activities. Several techniques with subtle variations have been described, with each having its own theoretical advantages, but few reports have provided clear guidelines that dictate the pathways of an algorithmic approach to OCD management. Some evidence shows that larger lesions and those in skeletally mature patients may be slower or less likely to heal, which can be important for setting expectations with families and ensuring close monitoring in the postoperative period. Meticulous preoperative assessment of MR images and arthroscopic assessment for signs of instability in OCD lesions are critical for proper treatment selection, because unstable lesions generally require more advanced techniques other than isolated drilling, such as drilling with fixation and the possible addition of debridement of the backside of the lesion and/or bone grafting. The systematic review performed by Gunton and colleagues[7] provides a comparative overview of the patient-oriented outcome measures, radiographic healing rates and times, and complications of the transarticular and retroarticular techniques. Importantly, both techniques showed healing rates around 90% occurring at a mean of 4 to 6 months, with no reported complications. However, better research methods, in the form of comparative, prospective studies in larger populations, are clearly needed to elucidate the relative benefits of different drilling techniques, and will be important for future treatment optimization for patients with OCD.

REFERENCES

1. Konig F. Ueber freie korper in den gelenken. Dtsch Z Chir 1887;27(90):109.
2. Kocher MS, Tucker R, Ganley TJ, et al. Management of osteochondritis dissecans of the knee: current concepts review. Am J Sports Med 2006;34(7):1181–91.
3. Flynn JM, Kocher MS, Ganley TJ. Osteochondritis dissecans of the knee. J Pediatr Orthop 2004;24(4):434–43.
4. Kocher M, Micheli L, Yaniv M, et al. Functional and radiographic outcome of juvenile osteochondritis dissecans of the knee treated with transarticular arthroscopic drilling. Am J Sports Med 2001;29(5):562–6.
5. Anderson A, Richards D, Pagnani MJ, et al. Antegrade drilling for osteochondritis dissecans of the knee. Arthroscopy 1997;13(3):319–24.
6. Aglietti P, Buzzi R, Bassi PB, et al. Arthroscopic drilling in juvenile osteochondritis dissecans of the medial femoral condyle. Arthroscopy 1994;10(3):286–91.
7. Gunton MJ, Carey JL, Shaw CR, et al. Drilling juvenile osteochondritis dissecans: retro- or transarticular? Clin Orthop Relat Res 2013;471(4):1144–51.
8. Boughanem J, Riaz R, Patel RM, et al. Functional and radiographic outcomes of juvenile osteochondritis dissecans of the knee treated with extra-articular retrograde drilling. Am J Sports Med 2011;39(10):2212–7.
9. Edmonds E, Albright J, Bastrom T, et al. Outcomes of extra-articular, intra-epiphyseal drilling for osteochondritis dissecans of the knee. J Pediatr Orthop 2010; 30(8):870–8.
10. Donaldson L, Wojtys E. Extraarticular drilling for stable osteochondritis dissecans in the skeletally immature knee. J Pediatr Orthop 2008;28(8):831–5.
11. Kawasaki K, Uchioa Y, Adachi N, et al. Drilling from the intercondylar area for treatment of osteochondritis dissecans of the knee joint. Knee 2003;10(3): 257–63.

The Knee
Internal Fixation Techniques for Osteochondritis Dissecans

Nathan L. Grimm, BS[a], Christopher K. Ewing, DO[b],
Theodore J. Ganley, MD[c],*

KEYWORDS

- Osteochondritis dissecans • Knee • Sports medicine • Fixation
- Skeletally immature

KEY POINTS

- The "stability" of an osteochondritis dissecans (OCD) lesion refers to the mechanical integrity of the lesion and an unstable lesion typically warrants surgical planning.
- Determining the physeal patency and stability of an OCD lesion is paramount to determining surgical intervention versus nonoperative, conservative treatment.
- The theoretical advantage of variable-pitch screw fixation for OCD lesions is decreased soft-tissue morbidity seen with the exiting Kirschner wire and articular cartilage morbidity seen with the head of a cannulated screw.
- Bioabsorbable products obviate a second surgery for hardware removal. However, there is a risk of device breakage, backing out, and elicitation of unwanted immune response.

INTRODUCTION

The decision to pursue surgical management of osteochondritis dissecans (OCD) in the athlete depends on multiple variables and should be a shared decision between the patient and surgeon. First and foremost, the patient's current quality of life, level of activity, sport, and goals should be assessed so that expectations are met for both parties. Following this, determining the stability of the OCD lesion is paramount.

There was no outside funding for this study.
The authors have nothing to disclose.
[a] Department of Orthopaedic Surgery, Duke University Medical Center, Box 3956, Durham, NC 27710, USA; [b] Department of Orthopaedics, Navy Medical Center San Diego, 34800 Bob Wilson Drive, San Diego, CA 92134, USA; [c] Department of Orthopaedics, Sports Medicine and Performance Center, The Children's Hospital of Philadelphia, 34th Street & Civic Center Boulevard, 2nd Floor, Wood Building, Philadelphia, PA 19104, USA
* Corresponding author.
E-mail address: ganley@email.chop.edu

Clin Sports Med 33 (2014) 313–319
http://dx.doi.org/10.1016/j.csm.2013.12.001
0278-5919/14/$ – see front matter © 2014 Elsevier Inc. All rights reserved.

Having an understanding of how stable the lesion is will help direct the surgeon down a path of conservative management versus surgical management.

The term "stability," in regards to OCD lesions, has been referred to as the mechanical integrity of the subchondral OCD lesion.[1] More specifically, an OCD lesion that is mobile, fragmented, or ex situ is thought to be unstable, and a lesion, which is immobile and in situ, is considered to be stable. The importance of this distinction is that it will help the surgeon and athletes avoid a potentially unnecessary or inappropriate surgery. Perhaps equally as important is the patency of the physis. Despite having an increased rate of OCD in young athletes,[2] it is well understood that juvenile osteochondritis dissecans (JOCD) typically has better outcomes than adult OCD. In 1985 Bernard Cahill[3] writes, "JOCD and OCD are distinct conditions. The former has a much more favorable prognosis than the latter."

Multiple classifications for predicting the stability of OCD lesions have been devised based on radiograph,[4,5] magnetic resonance imaging,[6–8] and arthroscopy.[7,9–12] The utility of classifications lies in their ability to predict whether a lesion is or will become unstable. This information is again useful for surgical decision-making and planning. It is important to remember that when planning surgical intervention of an OCD lesion the 4 key precepts described by Cahill[3] be considered: whenever possible restore the joint surface, enhance blood supply of the fragment, use rigid fixation where instability exists, and begin joint motion as soon as possible postoperatively.

The purpose of this article is to provide a detailed overview of the surgical options for internal fixation of OCD lesions (**Table 1**). The surgical techniques for internal fixation of OCD of the knee can be extrapolated to the treatment of OCD in other joints. In

Table 1
Methods of internal fixation for unstable OCD of the knee[a]

Method	Advantages	Disadvantages
Metallic devices		
Kirschner wire	Cost, availability, ease of placement	Exit site morbidity, lack of compression, need for removal, bending
Cannulated screws	Good fixation, multiple size options	Increased damage to articular surface from screw head, need for removal, backing out
Variable-pitch screws	Good fixation, "headless" counter-sinking	Possible need for removal
Bioabsorbable devices		
Pins/rods/pins	Size, planes of fixation, less stress shielding	Breakage, loss of fixation, foreign-body immune response
Screws	Good fixation, obviate hardware removal	Breakage, loss of fixation, foreign-body immune response
Biologic devices		
Mosaicplasty	Native tissue, graft across interface, obviate hardware removal	Possible donor site fracture, bone peg loosening, technically more challenging
Bone sticks	Native tissue, graft across interface, obviate hardware removal	Donor site morbidity, loss of fixation, technique in its infancy, technically more challenging

[a] Note: This list is not exhaustive and only includes those devices that historically have been used and studied most frequently.

addition, the methods of fixation described herein are typically indicated for fixation of unstable, salvageable lesions.

SURGICAL TECHNIQUES OF INTERNAL FIXATION
Screw Fixation

Variable-pitch and cannulated screws
Although originally described by Herbert and Fisher[13] for fixation of scaphoid fractures in1984, Wombwell and Nunley[14] describe its use in knee OCD lesions through an open arthrotomy and Thomson[15] describe its use in knee OCD lesions arthroscopically in 1987 (**Fig. 1**). More recently, Kouzelis and colleagues[16] reported successful fixation of unstable lesions in patients aged 14 to 26 using variable-pitch screw fixation. In this small series of 10 patients, with a mean follow-up of 27 months, radiographic union was observed in 9 of 10 patients and return to previous daily and sport activity was also seen in 9 of 10 patients.

In contrast to the variable-pitch screw, Cugat and colleagues[17] report on a small series of 14 patients (15 knees) with OCD lesions, all of whom participated in sports, using cannulated screws as a means of fixation (see **Fig. 1**). In this series there was a mean follow-up of 43 months and Cugat and colleagues[17] reported good or excellent results in 93% of this series with minimal complications. However, Thomson[15] reports the advantage of variable-pitch screw fixation is evidenced by the decreased soft tissue morbidity seen with Kirschner wire fixation and decreased articular cartilage morbidity seen with cannulated screw fixation.

Biologic Fixation

Mosaicplasty and bone sticks
Miniaci and Tytherleigh-Strong[18] report on a series of 20 patients (age range 12–27) with OCD of the knee who underwent autogenous osteochondral grafting (mosaic-plasty) technique. Similar to other reports using fixation with mosaicplasty,[19,20] the Miniaci and Tytherleigh-Strong[18] series showed excellent 1-year outcomes and a

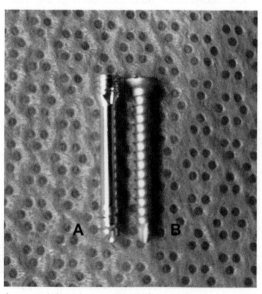

Fig. 1. Variable-pitch screw (A) and constant-pitch cannulated screw (B).

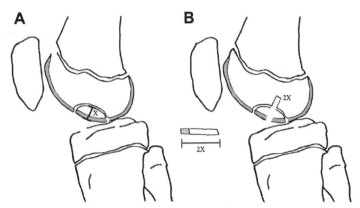

Fig. 2. (A) Depth of lesion at midpoint (X) and (B) length of bone plug and drill hole, which should be twice the length of midpoint depth (2X).

return to activity and sports. The caveat for successful fixation with this technique, as described by Miniaci and Tytherleigh-Strong, is that the graft must be long enough to pass at least far enough into the normal underlying subchondral bone as the distance it has passed through the lesion and across the interface (**Fig. 2**). Furthermore, the dimensions of osteochondral plugs harvested for this series of patients was 4.5 mm × 15 mm, respectively. This number was derived from calculations based on preoperative magnetic resonance imaging. The minimum length of the osteochondral plug can be derived by taking the midpoint of the widest section of the lesion and then simply doubling the depth of the lesion at the point.

Navarro and colleagues[21] describe an innovative technique in a series of 11 patients aged 11 to 20 years old with OCD of the knee and, although the level of activity was not specifically described, report that at least one patient in this series was an elite soccer player. This technique involves the use of autologous "bone sticks" harvested from the tibia medial to the tibial tubercle (**Fig. 3**A). Through a longitudinal incision, medial to the tibial tubercle, a microsaw is used to harvest several "bone sticks," which are subsequently used as a rigid biologic fixation for the OCD lesion (see **Fig. 3**B). With a mean follow-up of 48 months and satisfactory results in 90% of cases, Navarro and colleagues[21] state the advantages of this technique including obviation of large incisions or arthrotomy, solid fixation, and no need for hardware removal.

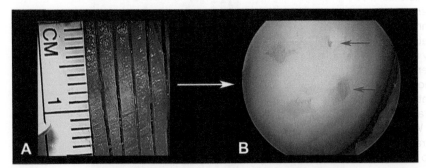

Fig. 3. (A) Bone sticks created with microsaw. (B) Placement of bone sticks through unstable lesion. (*Courtesy of* Ganley TJ, MD, Philadelphia PA.)

The advantage of these techniques lies in their ability to augment fixation through the formation of bone grafting across the interface of the progeny fragment and the parent bone. This fixation obviously cannot be achieved in the setting of metallic fixation. In addition, the use of such osteochondral plugs obviates the use of a second surgery for hardware removal. The caveat is that even with the theoretical advantages, reports of bone peg loosening, donor site fractures, and failure have been described.

Other

Kirschner wire, biodegradable rods/darts/pins

Anderson and colleagues[22] report good to excellent results in most cases using an interesting technique of autologous bone grafting and subsequent fragment fixation using Kirschner wires in a series of 16 patients (17 knees). Although this technique has several advantages including cost, availability, and ease of technique, there are disadvantages, such as lack of compression, a need for removal, bending of the wire, and exit site morbidity, which are not seen with other fixation devices. In addition, with the refinement of metallic screws and bioabsorbable fixation products, Kirschner wire seems to have lost favor.

Din and colleagues[23] reported on a series of 11 athletic patients with 12 OCD lesions of the knee, classified as Guhl[12] type I and II, using polylactide bioabsorbable pins (Intra Fix Smart Nails; Conmed-Linvatec, Tampere, Finland) for internal fixation. In this small series, Din and colleagues[23] report excellent outcomes in 8 of 12 knees and good outcomes in 4 of 12 knees using the Hughston rating scale. Furthermore, Din and colleagues claim that stabilization with the polylactide bioabsorbable pins allowed for an early return to sports.[5,24,25] However, several reports of loosening, breakage, and florid synovitis have been described.[26–29] It is also important to note that Kocher and colleagues[30] showed no statistically significant difference between healing outcomes seen between the use of bioabsorbable pins and tacks, metallic variable pitch screws, or partially threaded cannulated screws. The caveat for interpretation of this study however is the number of subjects for each group (between 3 and 11 subjects for each treatment arm).[30]

Preferred postoperative management

In the postoperative athlete who has undergone internal fixation of an unstable OCD lesion, the counseling on adherence to rehabilitation and activity restriction is paramount. The success of the fixation and outcome will depend not only on the surgery performed but also on the compliance of the athlete during this crucial period. A candid discussion of the importance of this convalescence period is discussed with the athlete as well as the athlete's family, when appropriate. During the postoperative period, following internal fixation, the authors prefer placing the patient in a knee immobilizer or hinged knee brace for 4 to 6 weeks to facilitate compliance and eliminate shearing forces. The brace is kept in full extension and the affected lower extremity is kept non-weight-bearing for a period of 4 weeks. To maintain motion patients are permitted to unlock the hinged brace or remove the brace for heel slides or a passive motion machine for a few minutes each day from the immediate postoperative period until the knee brace is removed. Patients are typically allowed to bear weight with the brace locked in extension from postoperative week 4 to week 6.

With the patient restricted from athletic involvement, gentle physical therapy (eg, straight leg raises and isometric exercises) is initiated shortly after fixation. Follow-up radiographs are taken at 3 months postoperatively. If evidence of healing is apparent, a return to "sportlike" activity is initiated and gradually increased over the course of 4 to 6 more weeks. A return to sport is then initiated with restrictions to lower intensity during practice and games with a gradual increase in intensity at the patient's discretion.

SUMMARY

As pointed out in **Table 1**, many fixation techniques are currently used and each has its advantages and disadvantages. The evolution of fixation devices has progressed from smooth pins to flat head and variable pitch screws. Given the low incidence of osteochondritis dissecans further high quality comparative multicenter study of fixation techniques is indicated. While there is no single universal fixation technique, clinicians should be facile with different techniques to accommodate for the unique size, depth and individual characteristics of each lesion. Following the principles of lesion preparation and mastering different techniques will allow for optimal treatment of osteochondritis dissecans lesions.

REFERENCES

1. Mesgarzadeh M, Sapega AA, Bonakdarpour A, et al. Osteochondritis dissecans: analysis of mechanical stability with radiography, scintigraphy, and MR imaging. Radiology 1987;165(3):775–80.
2. Cahill BR. Current concepts review. Osteochondritis dissecans. J Bone Joint Surg Am 1997;79(3):471–2.
3. Cahill B. Treatment of juvenile osteochondritis dissecans and osteochondritis dissecans of the knee. Clin Sports Med 1985;4(2):367–84.
4. Berndt AL, Harty M. Transchondral fractures (osteochondritis dissecans) of the talus. J Bone Joint Surg Am 1959;41:988–1020.
5. Hughston JC. Hergenroeder PT, Courtenay BG. Osteochondritis dissecans of the femoral condyles. J Bone Joint Surg Am 1984;66(9):1340–8.
6. Bohndorf K. Osteochondritis (osteochondrosis) dissecans: a review and new MRI classification. Eur Radiol 1998;8(1):103–12.
7. Dipaola JD, Nelson DW, Colville MR. Characterizing osteochondral lesions by magnetic resonance imaging. Arthroscopy 1991;7(1):101–4.
8. Kramer J, Stiglbauer R, Engel A, et al. MR contrast arthrography (MRA) in osteochondrosis dissecans. J Comput Assist Tomogr 1992;16(2):254–60.
9. ICRS Cartilage injury evaluation package. Developed during ICRS 2000 Standards Workshop at Schloss Münchenwiler. Switzerland, 2000. Available at: http://www.cartilage.org/_files/contentmanagement/ICRS_evaluation.pdf. Accessed May 27, 2013.
10. Baumgarten TE, Andrews JR, Satterwhite YE. The arthroscopic classification and treatment of osteochondritis dissecans of the capitellum. Am J Sports Med 1998; 26(4):520–3.
11. Ewing JW, Voto SJ. Arthroscopic surgical management of osteochondritis dissecans of the knee. Arthroscopy 1988;4(1):37–40.
12. Guhl JF. Arthroscopic treatment of osteochondritis dissecans. Clin Orthop Relat Res 1982;167:65–74.
13. Herbert TJ, Fisher WE. Management of the fractured scaphoid using a new bone screw. J Bone Joint Surg Br 1984;66(1):114–23.
14. Wombwell JH, Nunley JA. Compressive fixation of osteochondritis dissecans fragments with Herbert screws. J Orthop Trauma 1987;1(1):74–7.
15. Thomson NL. Osteochondritis dissecans and osteochondral fragments managed by Herbert compression screw fixation. Clin Orthop Relat Res 1987; 224:71–8.

16. Kouzelis A, Plessas S, Papadopoulos AX, et al. Herbert screw fixation and reverse guided drillings, for treatment of types III and IV osteochondritis dissecans. Knee Surg Sports Traumatol Arthrosc 2006;14(1):70–5.

17. Cugat R, Garcia M, Cusco X, et al. Osteochondritis dissecans: a historical review and its treatment with cannulated screws. Arthroscopy 1993;9(6):675–84.

18. Miniaci A, Tytherleigh-Strong G. Fixation of unstable osteochondritis dissecans lesions of the knee using arthroscopic autogenous osteochondral grafting (mosaicplasty). Arthroscopy 2007;23(8):845–51.

19. Berlet GC, Mascia A, Miniaci A. Treatment of unstable osteochondritis dissecans lesions of the knee using autogenous osteochondral grafts (mosaicplasty). Arthroscopy 1999;15(3):312–6.

20. Kobayashi T, Fujikawa K, Oohashi M. Surgical fixation of massive osteochondritis dissecans lesion using cylindrical osteochondral plugs. Arthroscopy 2004;20(9):981–6.

21. Navarro R, Cohen M, Filho MC, et al. The arthroscopic treatment of osteochondritis dissecans of the knee with autologous bone sticks. Arthroscopy 2002;18(8):840–4.

22. Anderson AF, Lipscomb AB, Coulam C. Antegrade curettement, bone grafting and pinning of osteochondritis dissecans in the skeletally mature knee. Am J Sports Med 1990;18(3):254–61.

23. Din R, Annear P, Scaddan J. Internal fixation of undisplaced lesions of osteochondritis dissecans in the knee. J Bone Joint Surg Br 2006;88(7):900–4.

24. Lipscomb PR Jr, Lipscomb PR Sr, Bryan RS. Osteochondritis dissecans of the knee with loose fragments. Treatment by replacement and fixation with readily removed pins. J Bone Joint Surg Am 1978;60(2):235–40.

25. Smillie IS. Treatment of osteochondritis dissecans. J Bone Joint Surg Br 1957;39(2):248–60.

26. Dervin GF, Keene GC, Chissell HR. Biodegradable rods in adult osteochondritis dissecans of the knee. Clin Orthop Relat Res 1998;356:213–21.

27. Friden T, Rydholm U. Severe aseptic synovitis of the knee after biodegradable internal fixation. A case report. Acta Orthop Scand 1992;63(1):94–7.

28. Scioscia TN, Giffin JR, Allen CR, et al. Potential complication of bioabsorbable screw fixation for osteochondritis dissecans of the knee. Arthroscopy 2001;17(2):E7.

29. Tuompo P, Arvela V, Partio EK, et al. Osteochondritis dissecans of the knee fixed with biodegradable self-reinforced polyglycolide and polylactide rods in 24 patients. Int Orthop 1997;21(6):355–60.

30. Kocher MS, Czarnecki JJ, Andersen JS, et al. Internal fixation of juvenile osteochondritis dissecans lesions of the knee. Am J Sports Med 2007;35(5):712–8.

Salvage Techniques in Osteochondritis Dissecans

John D. Polousky, MD[a],*, Jay Albright, MD[b]

KEYWORDS

- Osteochondritis dissecans lesion • Osteochondral allografts
- Osteochondritis dissecans (OCD) • Osteochondral allograft
- Autologous chondrocyte implantation • Cartilage • Salvage
- Autologous cartilage implantation

KEY POINTS

- Large articular cartilage defects caused by osteochondritis dissecans pose a challenging problem for the patient and orthopedic surgeon.
- Although clinical results of simple excision and debridement of unsalvageable lesions provide good symptomatic relief in the short-term, those good early results deteriorate over time.
- Autologous cartilage implantation and fresh osteochondral allografts have demonstrated good clinical results in long-term studies for the salvage of large cartilage defects.
- There are also promising new technologies on the horizon that may reduce the need for multiple procedures while providing an equivalent clinical result.

INTRODUCTION

The central objective in the treatment of any osteochondritis dissecans (OCD) lesion is to preserve the native articular cartilage and bone. Unfortunately, there are those cases that either fail to heal despite appropriate treatment or present in such a deteriorated state that primary fixation is not possible. This situation is generally determined by the condition of the progeny fragment. If the progeny has comminuted into multiple small fragments or is incongruous with the donor site, or the articular cartilage is excessively deteriorated, primary fixation may not be the most viable option. In the case of an unsalvageable fragment, the surgeon is faced with several options, which are discussed in this article.

---

[a] The Rocky Mountain Youth Sports Medicine Institute, 14000 East Arapahoe Road, Centennial, CO 80111, USA; [b] Children's Hospital Colorado, 13123 East 16th Avenue, Aurora, CO 80045, USA
* Corresponding author.
E-mail address: johnpolousky@msn.com

Clin Sports Med 33 (2014) 321–333
http://dx.doi.org/10.1016/j.csm.2014.01.004
0278-5919/14/$ – see front matter © 2014 Elsevier Inc. All rights reserved.
sportsmed.theclinics.com

DEBRIDEMENT/MICROFRACTURE/OSTEOCHONDRAL AUTOGRAFT TRANSPLANTATIONS

Debridement

The simplest solution to the unsalvageable OCD lesion is excision of the progeny fragment with debridement of the donor site. In the short-term, this approach has demonstrated good clinical results.[1–7] Unfortunately, these initial good results seem to deteriorate over time.[8,9] Murray and colleagues[10] demonstrated that 71% of patients who had undergone excision showed early degenerative changes on radiographs, despite having good subjective knee scores. Wright and colleagues[11] showed that two-thirds of patients had fair to poor radiographic results on the Hughston radiographic rating scale for OCD at an average of 9 years of follow-up. Finally, Anderson and Pagnani[12] found that most patients treated with excision scored poorly on both International Knee Documentation Committee (IKDC) and Hughston radiographic scores at a mean of 9 years of follow-up.

The above studies seem to indicate that, in the short-term, the symptoms of OCD are caused by the mechanical irritation of the unstable fragments. However, in the long-term, the poor results are more related to the loss of articular cartilage and the degenerative changes, which occur more slowly. Therefore, one could conclude that every attempt should be made to either repair the native bone and cartilage or fill the defect to produce a congruent articular surface.

Marrow Stimulation

The techniques of marrow stimulation have taken multiple forms: abrasion arthroplasty, drilling, and microfracture. The common principle between these techniques is the stimulation of marrow elements to produce fibrocartilage. Unlike hyaline cartilage, fibrocartilage has a high proportion of type 1 collagen as opposed to type 2 collagen. Fibrocartilage also lacks the intricate structural organization of hyaline cartilage. These factors may contribute to decreased durability when compared with techniques that use hyaline cartilage. Gudas and colleagues[13] conducted a prospective, randomized trial comparing osteochondral autograft transplantation with microfracture, specifically for the treatment of juvenile OCD. After the first year, both groups were equivalent, demonstrating significant clinical improvement over their preoperative state. However, the results of the microfracture group deteriorated over time. At 4 years, 41% of the microfracture group failed. There were no failures in the osteochondral autograft group. This difference was statistically significant.

Osteochondral Autograft Transplantation

Osteochondral autograft transplantation[13] offers an attractive option for replacing the osteochondral defect left by an unsalvageable OCD because it addresses both the bone and the cartilage deficiency with a single graft. As mentioned above, good results have been reported when used in cases of knee OCDs.[13] The obvious limitation of the technique is the surface area of donor cartilage available. Larger defects require multiple small grafts placed in a mosaic technique. When the mosaic technique is used, fibrocartilage fills the space between the grafts, which may have an impact on durability. Also, placing many small grafts can lead to incongruity of the articular surface. Poor results have been reported when osteochondral autografting is used in lesions greater than 6 cm^2.[14,15]

FRESH OSTEOCHONDRAL ALLOGRAFT

Osteochondral allograft transplantation has been proposed for large, unsalvageable OCD lesions for nearly 60 years.[4] Approximately 40 years ago, several centers in North

America began osteochondral allograft transplantation programs.[16] These centers both procured and transplanted the tissue. The principle of fresh osteochondral allograft transplantation is to replace a very focal area of disease in an otherwise healthy joint with intact, living hyaline cartilage. The only portion of the graft tissue requiring healing is the donor bone to the host bone, which occurs via creeping substitution. The donor chondrocytes remain viable, maintaining the matrix, and are not replaced by host cells.[17]

Unlike solid organ transplantation, cartilage transplantation seems to generate a negligible host immunologic response, making pharmacologic suppression unnecessary. This lack of response seems to be related to the small number of living cells in the graft, as well as the protection offered by the chondral matrix. Langer and Gross[18] demonstrated, in both rat and rabbit models, that transplantation of chondrocytes in an intact matrix produced no host cellular immune response. In contrast, when either chondrocytes without matrix or cartilage shavings were transplanted, a host cell-mediated immune response was generated. Williams and colleagues[16] demonstrated no immune rejection in retrieval specimens. These grafts had failed for a variety of reasons. However, there was no histologic evidence that a host immune response played a role.

SAFETY

The transfer of fresh osteochondral allografts transplants living chondrocytes from one human to another; therefore, tissue procurement is a critical step in the process. A need for rapid turnaround to preserve living tissue must be balanced with the safety of the recipient. Allograft tissue transplantation is widely used on orthopedic surgery and disease transmission is exceedingly rare.[19]

Chondrocyte viability, cell density, and metabolic activity all significantly decrease, after 14 days from harvest. However, the glycosaminoglycan content and biomechanical properties of the cartilage are maintained after 28 days of storage.[20]

Currently, fresh osteochondral allografts are procured and stored according to the American Association of Tissue Banks regulations. They are recovered within 24 hours of donor expiration and stored in culture medium at 4°C until implantation. The grafts are held for 14 days for medical history review, serologic testing, and culture. After 14 days, assuming negative medical history, serology, and culture, the grafts are released for implantation with an expiration date at 28 days postprocurement.[21]

SURGICAL TECHNIQUE

Preoperatively, the donor and recipient are size matched based on plain radiographs, magnetic resonance imaging, or computed tomographic scan. The dowel and shell techniques are commonly used in the setting of chondral defects.[17,22]

The dowel technique is used for smaller lesions. This technique requires a set of specialized reamers to achieve a press fit between the donor bone and recipient site. The proper diameter of the required graft is determined. A guide pin is placed through the center of the sizer with the sizer in even contact with the articular surface; this step ensures that the trajectory of the guide pin is perpendicular to the articular surface. The guide pin is left in place and the edge of the area to be prepared is scored to prevent peeling of the surrounding cartilage during reaming. The corresponding recipient site reamer is selected and the site is reamed over the guide pin until healthy, bleeding subchondral bone is encountered, generally 8 to 15 mm from the chondral surface. The 12-o'clock position is marked on the articular surface. Depth measurements are taken and recorded at the 3-, 6-, 9-, and 12-o'clock positions. Attention is now turned to the donor condyle. The corresponding anatomic area is identified to match the contour of the recipient as closely as possible. A guide pin can be placed through the sizer to assist with maintaining a perpendicular trajectory with the reamer if necessary. Again, the cartilage of the donor is scored; the 12-o'clock position is marked on the graft, and it is cut with the dowel reamer. The graft is then removed from the donor condyle with a sagittal saw, taking care to preserve the appropriate depth. When the dowel is free, it is trimmed to the appropriate depths at the marked clock positions. Pulsatile irrigation is used to remove marrow elements from the donor bone and the graft is placed. Generally, the graft is secure with a press fit. If further fixation is desired, small, absorbable pins may be used.

Using multiple grafts, the "snowman" technique can increase the area covered by the dowel graft technique. The second graft is placed interdigitating with the first graft. Before reaming into the first graft, it is important for the surgeon to fix the graft temporarily with 2 small k-wires to prevent displacement during reaming.

The shell technique is generally used for larger lesions. Once the lesion is exposed, it is debrided to form a simple geometric shape. Approximately 2 to 3 mm of subchondral bone is removed from the recipient site to expose healthy host bone. Autogenous bone grafting may be performed for large, deep bony defects. Once the defect is sculpted into a simple shape with a smooth flat base, a template can be drawn noting the lengths of the sides and depth at each edge of the defect. The surface contour of the donor and recipient condyle is matched. Once the area of best fit is localized, the graft is cut using a small sagittal saw. Multiple trials and trimmings are usually needed to refine the fit of the graft. Once the appropriate fit is achieved with the graft either flush or slightly recessed, the graft is irrigated with pulsatile lavage and implanted. The graft is then secured with a combination of interference fit and small, absorbable, polydiaxanone pins.

Postoperative care for both methods consists of immediate range of motion to allow for cartilage nutrition. Weight-bearing is generally protected for 6 to 12 weeks with resumption of full activity at 4 to 6 months (**Figs. 1–3**).[22]

CLINICAL RESULTS

Multiple authors have reported good results using fresh osteochondral allografts for the reconstruction of posttraumatic cartilage defects about the knee.[17,23,24] Emmerson and colleagues[22] reported the long-term results of fresh osteochondral allografting in a group of patients with the specific diagnosis of OCD. The study group included

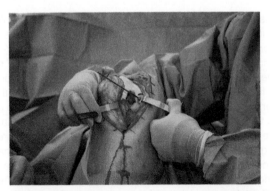

Fig. 1. The guide pin is placed in the center in the lesion, perpendicular to the articular surface.

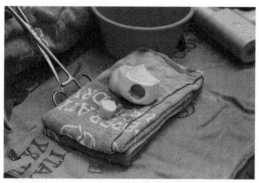

Fig. 2. The graft is removed after cutting with the dowel reamer.

66 knees in 64 patients. The mean age was 28.8 years. The mean follow-up was 7.7 years. The authors reported 72% good or excellent results with a 15% reoperation rate. Factors associated with reoperation were older age and larger lesions. The 5-year survivorship was 91%.

Unlike posttraumatic chondral defects, which often have associated ligamentous instability and bony malalignment, OCD lesions are generally a focal defect in an otherwise healthy knee belonging to a younger patient. If associated pathologic abnormality is present, such as coronal plane malalignment or ligamentous deficiency, it should be addressed in conjunction with osteochondral allografting procedures.[17,22,25–27]

FUTURE DIRECTIONS IN ALLOGRAFT CARTILAGE SALVAGE

Over the past several years, 2 new commercially available products have become available for treating articular cartilage defects with morselized autograft or juvenile allograft cartilage. CAIS (Cartilage Autograft Implantation System; Depuy, Raynham, MA, USA) uses cartilage autograft. DeNovo NT (ISTO, St. Louis, MO, USA) uses juvenile donor allograft cartilage. Both systems suspend the cartilage in a delivery medium, allowing a single-stage procedure for filling the chondral defect. Laboratory and animal studies have demonstrated migration of the chondrocytes to form hyaline-like cartilage in the defect.[28] At the time of writing this article, there are 2 published articles on the treatments of full-thickness chondral defects in the knee,

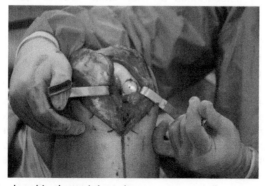

Fig. 3. The graft is placed in the recipient site.

specifically the patella, with particulated juvenile cartilage.[29,30] Both retrospective studies demonstrate promising early results on both magnetic resonance imaging evaluation and patient-oriented outcomes. Good results have also been published using this technology for chondral defects in the talus.[31–33] Further studies are necessary to determine if this technology produces good long-term outcomes for large chondral lesions associated with OCD.

AUTOLOGOUS CARTILAGE IMPLANTATION
History

Smith[34] was the first to isolate and grow chondrocytes in a culture medium in 1965; however, Chesterman and Smith[35] had limited success injecting these cells into the rabbit knee. In 1987, 3 years after Peterson[36] introduced the periosteal flap to seal the cells into a rabbit defect model, Peterson and colleagues[37,38] began the human implantation using this technique. Since then, over 10,000 procedures have been done throughout the world. Most recently, there are up to 20-year follow-up studies demonstrating good durability and maintenance of function in up to 75% of patients treated. Those that fail tend to do so within the first 2 years.

Histology

The main goal of any cartilage restoration or even salvage technique is to obtain the best and most durable tissue that as closely resembles natural cartilage structure and architecture as possible. Autologous cartilage implantation (ACI) histologically can be described as having hyaline-type cartilage or hyaline-like cartilage. The best specimens at biopsy have been documented to resemble closely normal hyaline cartilage. On the opposite end of the spectrum, some biopsies specimens appear to be fibrocartilage with some type II hyaline cartilage mixed in. Sixty-five percent of patients with macroscopically normal repairs have hyaline or hyaline-like cartilage at reoperation, whereas only 25% of those with macroscopically abnormal repairs at repeat surgery have type 2 hyaline or hyaline-like cartilage.[39,40]

Indications

The use of ACI or transplantation has been indicated for lesions between 2 and 16 cm^2 in size. It is typically used as a salvage technique for contained, irreparable lesions from osteochondritis dissecans or osteochondral injuries, either acute fracture or chronic lesions such as focal osteoarthritis. A noncontained lesion is a relative indication and not a contraindication; however, the use of this technique in kissing or diffuse lesions such as in osteoarthritis or rheumatoid arthritis lesions is still under investigation.[37,41–44]

Surgical Technique

ACI is a 2-step technique, which requires 2 anesthetics. The first surgery is an arthroscopic evaluation to (1) determine if a patient is a candidate for ACI and (2) address any other intra-articular pathologic abnormality such as meniscal tears. Noninjured cartilage is then biopsied all the way to subchondral bone from a less needed area of the knee: the superomedial aspect of the trochlear groove, the superolateral aspect of the trochlear groove, or the intercondylar notch. All locations have potential drawbacks of removing cartilage from these locations, but after 1200 biopsies, no significant morbidity has been reported.[40,45] The cartilage is sent in a special container to a laboratory where the cells are separated, processed, and multiplied to produce 10 to 15 times more cells. This process can take as little as 2 to 4 weeks.[36]

A second procedure is then performed similar to that described by Peterson[44] in 2002. The approach is predicated by the location of the lesion. A sufficient arthrotomy needs to be made to allow for easy exposure to the entire lesion and should be determined during preoperative planning. All concomitant surgery can be performed as well, such as correction of malalignment or other intra-articular pathologic abnormality.[46] Once the lesion is exposed, creating vertical walls around the entire lesion, removing any undermined, fray, fissured, or otherwise unhealthy cartilage should be done to prepare the lesion.

Frequently larger OCD lesions have significant subchondral bone loss. Subchondral bone defects with a depth greater than 6 to 8 mm should be bone grafted. The bed is prepared by removing the sclerotic bone rim with a bur or curette, drilling multiple tunnels for bleed tracts, and then filling the defect with cancellous bone from a local source such as Gerdy tubercle or the iliac crest. Next a template of the lesion is made with sterile paper or foil and a periosteal flap is obtained. The proximal medial tibia is often used as a harvest site for this or, if concomitant osteotomies are being done, the harvest can be done at this location. After exposure and marking of the fibrous side of the periosteum is completed, the template is used and a 1- to 2-mm larger periosteal flap is cut sharply down to bone. A small periosteal elevator is then used to remove the flap carefully, trying to avoid holes or penetration of the flap. Once the flap is removed, the fibrous side (marked) needs to be kept moist. The periosteal flap, with the cambium side up toward the joint, is then sutured over the graft. A 6-0 absorbable suture is ideal and is sewn in a figure-of-8 fashion, starting at the 4 corners of the lesion, leaving the knots over the flap as it is tied to the base of the cartilage defect. Sutures are then filled in, tensioning the flap in an alternating fashion from side to side, until a small area is left open. Fibrin glue is placed into the space between the fibrous layer and the bone graft and pressurized with the surgeon's digit for 1 minute. The tourniquet should be released to confirm that this closure remains bloodless.

If no bone loss exists, then curettes should be used to prepare the bone bed, avoiding penetrating the subchondral bone but removing the calcified cartilage layer if present. A small amount of fibrin glue compressed into the prepared bone bed can be used to maintain a bloodless substrate for the grafting. Whether or not bone grafting was needed, a periosteal or synthetic flap is now needed to cover the superficial portion of the defect. The flap is obtained in the same fashion as above, using the template of the lesion size. This periosteal flap is then sutured in the same sequence with the cambium layer down or facing the bone and the fibrous layer facing the joint. A small opening is left at the most superior portion of the flap for insertion of the autologous cells. Fibrin glue is placed in the intervals between the sutures to make the construct watertight. Using a soft plastic catheter, a syringe is used to slowly inject saline into the defect through the small opening. Once it is confirmed that the construct is watertight, the saline is removed, and the cells are then injected, withdrawing the catheter as the cells are injected. The final suture is placed along with fibrin glue to complete the grafting. The knee is then closed in layers.

Postoperatively, the knee is braced and left still for around 6 to 8 hours to allow the graft to set. A continuous passive motion device or passive motion is started 0° to 60° postoperative day 1 for the first 4 weeks. A range of motion of 0° to 90° is then allowed until 6 weeks. Partial weight-bearing status is allowed immediately, but the amount is determined based on size, location of lesion, as well as the concomitant procedures performed. Return to full weight-bearing typically is allowable at between 6 and 12 weeks postoperatively depending on factors mentioned above. Running is discouraged until 6 to 9 months postoperatively.

Results

Autologous chondrocyte implantation has some of the longest follow-up of any of these salvage procedures. The results at medium range follow-up (10+ years) have been mixed with anywhere from 65% to 90% good to excellent results in the best hands doing this procedure, with results favorable to mosaicplasty in one study at 10 years.[40,47–49] However, the efficacy and safety of ACI in the pediatric population has not been established because of the paucity of quality research on children less than 18 years of age.[50] One recent study in children and adolescents[51] showed that ACI done in the younger patient (18 ± 2.3 years) shows different rates of expression of cartilage-specific makers compared with patients in the older group (23 years old) but the study was neither truly an adolescent or pediatric population nor a longitudinal outcome/efficacy study.

Complications

Most complications seem to be related to the periosteal flap from overgrowth, to delamination, to arthrofibrosis. When less than 1 cm of the lesion is delaminated, it is recommended to remove that piece only; however, if it is more, removal of the entire piece may be called for. Early therapy and range-of-motion exercises seem to be the best for preventing arthrofibrosis.[36]

MATRIX-INDUCED AUTOLOGOUS CARTILAGE IMPLANTATION

Matrix-induced autologous cartilage implantation (MACI) is considered, along with other similar collagen scaffolding or delivery mechanisms, to potentially be the next generation of cartilage regenerative technologies. Although none of the scaffolding systems are yet available in the United States, they have been used for 10 years or more in Europe and other countries. All of these technologies either use a collagen matrix that is mixed with the autologous chondrocytes harvested and processed similarly to the ACI technique or rely on marrow stimulation to supply the cells. MACI is significantly different from ACI in that the cartilage cells are being multiplied and then impregnated into a cartilage matrix before the implantation process, where the cells are injected free floating under the flap during ACI.[52–54]

SURGICAL TECHNIQUE

Depending on the size and location of the defect to be grafted, the ease of use of a more solid matrix lends itself to arthroscopic implantation or open implantation. During the surgery, the cartilage defect is prepared similarly to preparation of the defect in ACI, preparing the defect down to the calcified cartilage without penetration of the subchondral bone. The cartilage edges are prepared in as vertical stable edges as possible. The cartilage implant is then trimmed to match the lesion as close to exact as possible. The implant is then placed with the cell-seeded side facing the subchondral bone and fixed in place with fibrin glue, taking time to ensure the graft does not protrude out of the lesion. When the security of the implant is questionable, uncontained or large lesions, suture anchors, or simple suture fixation may be necessary with bioabsorbable suture.[55]

Postoperative protocol is similar to ACI in that the goals are the same to restore motion, strength, and coordination but to protect the integrity of the graft as it matures and heals. Continuous passive motion (CPM) is also used to attempt to increase synthesis of cartilage. Protected weight-bearing for 8 to 12 weeks is customary; however, the Australian experience with a randomized prospective trial has shown an accelerated rehabilitation protocol to be as effective.[55–57]

There is a growing literature in the world of MACI and its effectiveness for treating full-thickness cartilage defects when compared with other methods. Basad and colleagues[58] compared MACI with microfracture and showed significant improvements in outcomes. Bentley and colleagues[48] have also shown it to be superior to mosaicplasty in their hands, whereas Bartlett and colleagues[59] did not find a difference between MACI and ACI at 12 months. All of these studies are short-term and further research and long-term outcomes are needed; however, there is promise that these technologies as they advance will move us closer to helping patients even more.

FUTURE DIRECTIONS IN CELL-BASED CARTILAGE SALVAGE

In the United States, one new direction in cartilage salvage that is similar in concept to MACI using marrow stimulation or another source of stem or mesenchymal cells mixed with scaffolding is BioCartilage (Arthrex, Inc., Naples, FL),[60] an allograft technique that uses platelet-rich plasma mixed with an allogenic dehydrated, micronized cartilage implanted into the defect in a one-stage procedure. The mesenchymal stem cells are provided to populate the scaffold through microfracture of the subchondral bone and propagate chondrogenesis.[61] Although available currently and having passed initial studies on safety of use in humans after a 2-year follow-up study,[62] no other human studies are available on the outcomes of this technique. Its low cost and single-stage procedure make it an attractive option, especially with the animal and early nonrandomized results; however, time will tell whether this is a truly viable option as more head-to-head research is performed.

SUMMARY

Large articular cartilage defects caused by OCD pose a challenge for the patient and orthopedic surgeon. Although clinical results of simple excision and debridement of unsalvageable lesions are good symptomatic relief in the short-term, those good early results deteriorate over time. ACI and fresh osteochondral allografts have demonstrated good clinical results in long-term studies for the salvage of large cartilage defects. There are also promising new technologies on the horizon that may reduce the need for multiple procedures while providing an equivalent clinical result.

REFERENCES

1. Denoncourt PM, Patel D, Dimakopoulos P. Arthroscopy update #1. Treatment of osteochondrosis dissecans of the knee by arthroscopic curettage, follow-up study. Orthop Rev 1986;15(10):652–7.
2. Aglietti P, Ciardullo A, Giron F, et al. Results of arthroscopic excision of the fragment in the treatment of osteochondritis dissecans of the knee. Arthroscopy 2001;17(7):741–6.
3. Linden B. Osteochondritis dissecans of the femoral condyles: a long-term follow-up study. J Bone Joint Surg Am 1977;59(6):769–76.
4. Smillie IS. Treatment of osteochondritis dissecans. J Bone Joint Surg Br 1957; 39-B(2):248–60.
5. Schenck RC Jr, Goodnight JM. Osteochondritis dissecans. J Bone Joint Surg Am 1996;78(3):439–56.
6. Langenskiold A. Osteochondritis dissecans resulting from cartilage fractures due to trauma in early childhood. Duodecim 1955;71(1–2):232–9 [in Finnish].

7. Rehbein F. The origin of osteochondritis dissecans. Langenbecks Arch Klin Chir Ver Dtsch Z Chir 1950;265(1):69–114 [in Undetermined Language].

8. Cahill BR. Osteochondritis dissecans of the knee: treatment of juvenile and adult forms. J Am Acad Orthop Surg 1995;3(4):237–47.

9. Michael JW, Wurth A, Eysel P, et al. Long-term results after operative treatment of osteochondritis dissecans of the knee joint-30 year results. Int Orthop 2008; 32(2):217–21.

10. Murray JR, Chitnavis J, Dixon P, et al. Osteochondritis dissecans of the knee; long-term clinical outcome following arthroscopic debridement. Knee 2007; 14(2):94–8.

11. Wright RW, McLean M, Matava MJ, et al. Osteochondritis dissecans of the knee: long-term results of excision of the fragment. Clin Orthop Relat Res 2004;(424): 239–43.

12. Anderson AF, Pagnani MJ. Osteochondritis dissecans of the femoral condyles. Long-term results of excision of the fragment. Am J Sports Med 1997;25(6): 830–4.

13. Gudas R, Simonaityte R, Cekanauskas E, et al. A prospective, randomized clinical study of osteochondral autologous transplantation versus microfracture for the treatment of osteochondritis dissecans in the knee joint in children. J Pediatr Orthop 2009;29(7):741–8.

14. Horas U, Pelinkovic D, Herr G, et al. Autologous chondrocyte implantation and osteochondral cylinder transplantation in cartilage repair of the knee joint. A prospective, comparative trial. J Bone Joint Surg Am 2003;85-A(2): 185–92.

15. Wang CJ. Treatment of focal articular cartilage lesions of the knee with autogenous osteochondral grafts. A 2- to 4-year follow-up study. Arch Orthop Trauma Surg 2002;122(3):169–72.

16. Williams SK, Amiel D, Ball ST, et al. Analysis of cartilage tissue on a cellular level in fresh osteochondral allograft retrievals. Am J Sports Med 2007;35(12): 2022–32.

17. Bugbee WD, Convery FR. Osteochondral allograft transplantation. Clin Sports Med 1999;18(1):67–75.

18. Langer F, Gross AE. Immunogenicity of allograft articular cartilage. J Bone Joint Surg Am 1974;56(2):297–304.

19. Joyce MG, Greenwald AS, Boden S, et al. Musculoskeletal allograft tissue safety. AAOS Committee on patient safety-Committee on biological implants Workgroup findings. Presented at the 74th. Annual Meeting of the American Academy of Orthopaedic Surgeons, San Diego, CA. Feb 14–18, 2007.

20. Bentley G, Biant LC, Carrington RW, et al. A prospective, randomised comparison of autologous chondrocyte implantation versus mosaicplasty for osteochondral defects in the knee. J Bone Joint Surg Br 2003;85(2):223–30.

21. Banks AAoT. Available at: http://www.aatb.org. Accessed October 13, 2013.

22. Emmerson BC, Gortz S, Jamali AA, et al. Fresh osteochondral allografting in the treatment of osteochondritis dissecans of the femoral condyle. Am J Sports Med 2007;35(6):907–14.

23. Maury AC, Safir O, Heras FL, et al. Twenty-five-year chondrocyte viability in fresh osteochondral allograft. A case report. J Bone Joint Surg Am 2007;89(1): 159–65.

24. Shasha N, Krywulak S, Backstein D, et al. Long-term follow-up of fresh tibial osteochondral allografts for failed tibial plateau fractures. J Bone Joint Surg Am 2003;85-A(Suppl 2):33–9.

25. Pruthi S, Parnell SE, Thapa MM. Pseudointercondylar notch sign: manifestation of osteochondritis dissecans of the trochlea. Pediatr Radiol 2009;39(2):180–3.

26. Gross AE, Aubin P, Cheah HK, et al. A fresh osteochondral allograft alternative. J Arthroplasty 2002;17(4 Suppl 1):50–3.

27. Gross AE, Kim W, Las Heras F, et al. Fresh osteochondral allografts for posttraumatic knee defects: long-term followup. Clin Orthop Relat Res 2008;466(8): 1863–70.

28. Farr J, Cole BJ, Sherman S, et al. Particulated articular cartilage: CAIS and DeNovo NT. J Knee Surg 2012;25(1):23–9.

29. Bonner KF, Daner W, Yao JQ. 2-year postoperative evaluation of a patient with a symptomatic full-thickness patellar cartilage defect repaired with particulated juvenile cartilage tissue. J Knee Surg 2010;23(2):109–14.

30. Tompkins M, Hamann JC, Diduch DR, et al. Preliminary results of a novel single-stage cartilage restoration technique: particulated juvenile articular cartilage allograft for chondral defects of the patella. Arthroscopy 2013;29(10):1661–70.

31. Cerrato R. Particulated juvenile articular cartilage allograft transplantation for osteochondral lesions of the talus. Foot Ankle Clin 2013;18(1):79–87.

32. Coetzee JC, Giza E, Schon LC, et al. Treatment of osteochondral lesions of the talus with particulated juvenile cartilage. Foot Ankle Int 2013;34(9):1205–11.

33. Hatic SO 2nd, Berlet GC. Particulated juvenile articular cartilage graft (DeNovo NT Graft) for treatment of osteochondral lesions of the talus. Foot Ankle Spec 2010;3(6):361–4.

34. Smith AU. Survival of frozen chondrocytes isolated from cartilageof adult mammals. Nature 1965;205:782.

35. Chesterman PJ, Smith AU. Homotransplantation of articular cartilage and isolated chondrocytes. An experimental study in rabbits. J Bone Joint Surg Br 1968;50(1):184–97.

36. Peterson L. Technique of autologous chondrocyte implantation. Tech Knee Surg 2002;1(1):2–12.

37. Minas T, Von Keudell A, Bryant T, et al. The John Insall Award: a minimum 10-year outcome study of autologous chondrocyte implantation. Clin Orthop Relat Res 2013;472(1):41–51.

38. Peterson L, Vasiliadis HS, Brittberg M, et al. Autologous chondrocyte implantation: a long-term follow-up. Am J Sports Med 2010;38(6):1117–24.

39. Henderson I, Lavigne P, Valenzuela H, et al. Autologous chondrocyte implantation: superior biologic properties of hyaline cartilage repairs. Clin Orthop Relat Res 2007;455:253–61.

40. Peterson L, Brittberg M, Kiviranta I, et al. Autologous chondrocyte transplantation. Biomechanics and long-term durability. Am J Sports Med 2002;30(1):2–12.

41. Minas T. Autologous chondrocyte implantation for focal chondral defects of the knee. Clin Orthop Relat Res 2001;(Suppl 391):S349–61.

42. Minas T. Autologous chondrocyte implantation in the arthritic knee. Orthopedics 2003;26(9):945–7.

43. Noyes FR, Barber-Westin SD. Advanced patellofemoral cartilage lesions in patients younger than 50 years of age: is there an ideal operative option? Arthroscopy 2013;29(8):1423–36.

44. Peterson L, Minas T, Brittberg M, et al. Treatment of osteochondritis dissecans of the knee with autologous chondrocyte transplantation: results at two to ten years. J Bone Joint Surg Am 2003;85-A(Suppl 2):17–24.

45. LaPrade RF, Botker JC. Donor-site morbidity after osteochondral autograft transfer procedures. Arthroscopy 2004;20(7):e69–73.

46. Jacobi M, Wahl P, Bouaicha S, et al. Association between mechanical axis of the leg and osteochondritis dissecans of the knee: radiographic study on 103 knees. Am J Sports Med 2010;38(7):1425–8.

47. Vijayan S, Bartlett W, Bentley G, et al. Autologous chondrocyte implantation for osteochondral lesions in the knee using a bilayer collagen membrane and bone graft: a two- to eight-year follow-up study. J Bone Joint Surg Br 2012;94(4): 488–92.

48. Bentley G, Biant LC, Vijayan S, et al. Minimum ten-year results of a prospective randomised study of autologous chondrocyte implantation versus mosaicplasty for symptomatic articular cartilage lesions of the knee. J Bone Joint Surg Br 2012;94(4):504–9.

49. Moradi B, Schonit E, Nierhoff C, et al. First-generation autologous chondrocyte implantation in patients with cartilage defects of the knee: 7 to 14 years' clinical and magnetic resonance imaging follow-up evaluation. Arthroscopy 2012; 28(12):1851–61.

50. Kaszkin-Bettag M. Is autologous chondrocyte implantation (ACI) an adequate treatment option for repair of cartilage defects in paediatric patients? Drug Discov Today 2013;18(15–16):740–7.

51. Schmal H, Pestka JM, Salzmann G, et al. Autologous chondrocyte implantation in children and adolescents. Knee Surg Sports Traumatol Arthrosc 2013;21(3): 671–7.

52. Selmi TA, Verdonk P, Chambat P, et al. Autologous chondrocyte implantation in a novel alginate-agarose hydrogel: outcome at two years. J Bone Joint Surg Br 2008;90(5):597–604.

53. Trattnig S, Pinker K, Krestan C, et al. Matrix-based autologous chondrocyte implantation for cartilage repair with HyalograftC: two-year follow-up by magnetic resonance imaging. Eur J Radiol 2006;57(1):9–15.

54. Masri M, Lombardero G, Velasquillo C, et al. Matrix-encapsulation cell-seeding technique to prevent cell detachment during arthroscopic implantation of matrix-induced autologous chondrocytes. Arthroscopy 2007;23(8):877–83.

55. Jacobi M, Villa V, Magnussen RA, et al. MACI - a new era? Sports Med Arthrosc Rehabil Ther Technol 2011;3(1):10.

56. Ebert JR, Fallon M, Zheng MH, et al. A randomized trial comparing accelerated and traditional approaches to postoperative weightbearing rehabilitation after matrix-induced autologous chondrocyte implantation: findings at 5 years. Am J Sports Med 2012;40(7):1527–37.

57. Wondrasch B, Zak L, Welsch GH, et al. Effect of accelerated weightbearing after matrix-associated autologous chondrocyte implantation on the femoral condyle on radiographic and clinical outcome after 2 years: a prospective, randomized controlled pilot study. Am J Sports Med 2009;37(Suppl 1):88S–96S.

58. Basad E, Ishaque B, Bachmann G, et al. Matrix-induced autologous chondrocyte implantation versus microfracture in the treatment of cartilage defects of the knee: a 2-year randomised study. Knee Surg Sports Traumatol Arthrosc 2010;18(4):519–27.

59. Bartlett W, Skinner JA, Gooding CR, et al. Autologous chondrocyte implantation versus matrix-induced autologous chondrocyte implantation for osteochondral defects of the knee: a prospective, randomised study. J Bone Joint Surg Br 2005;87(5):640–5.

60. Abrams GD, Mall NA, Fortier LA, et al. BioCartilage: background and operative technique. Oper Tech Sports Med 2013;21(2):116–24.

61. Dhollander AA, De Neve F, Almqvist KF, et al. Autologous matrix-induced chondrogenesis combined with platelet-rich plasma gel: technical description and a five pilot patients report. Knee Surg Sports Traumatol Arthrosc 2011;19(4): 536–42.
62. Cole BJ, Farr J, Winalski CS, et al. Outcomes after a single-stage procedure for cell-based cartilage repair: a prospective clinical safety trial with 2-year follow-up. Am J Sports Med 2011;39(6):1170–9.

Future Treatment Strategies for Cartilage Repair

Roger Lyon, MD*, Xue-Cheng Liu, MD, PhD

KEYWORDS

- Cartilage repair • Tissue engineering • Cell therapy • Scaffolds • Growth factors

KEY POINTS

- The near future of cartilage repair will most likely involve refinement of current techniques along with incorporation of scientific advances in cartilage biology.
- With further development the implantation of a scaffold imbedded with stem cells and cartilage growth factors will likely be scientifically achievable and it is hoped could be made clinically viable and cost-effective.
- Ongoing research into cartilage repair should offer a single-stage surgical technique, which will replicate the structural characteristics of normal articular (hyaline) cartilage and incorporate onto bone.

INTRODUCTION

Cartilage repair remains a work in progress. Getting cartilage-like material to fill gaps in normal articular cartilage (AC) is possible with a variety of techniques. These replacement tissues have been analyzed for their various properties and bits and pieces of similarities with hyaline cartilage have been found. Cartilage substitutes and even benign neglect have been tried. All these modalities have met with variable success. Proponents of these methods tout the benefit of their specific approach but to date none of them would be considered a solution to cartilage defects for weight-bearing joints.

AC is an especially difficult tissue to induce and/or manufacture. It has a very complex structure and is almost inert with very little blood supply; its supporting cells are primarily for maintenance not repair, and therefore, matrix injury results in a very blunted and inadequate repair response.

Disclose Any Relationship: Each author certifies that he or she has no direct financial interest in the subject matter or materials discussed in the article or with a company making a competing product.

Department of Orthopaedic Surgery, Children's Hospital of Wisconsin, Medical College of Wisconsin, 9000 West Wisconsin Avenue, PO Box 1997, Pediatric Orthopaedics, Suite C360, Milwaukee, WI 53201, USA

* Corresponding author.
E-mail address: rlyon@chw.org

Clin Sports Med 33 (2014) 335–352
http://dx.doi.org/10.1016/j.csm.2013.12.003
0278-5919/14/$ – see front matter © 2014 Elsevier Inc. All rights reserved.

sportsmed.theclinics.com

Current strategies for repairing cartilage defects often report clinical success rates of 70% to 80% for pain relief and functional return. Fortunately clinical success is not solely correlated to reproduction of the form and attributes of AC. Many of the repair/replacement techniques compare themselves against the body's ability to repair itself. The tissue formed following microfracture has been popularized as the convenient cartilage repair tissue benchmark. Unfortunately none the techniques that seek to regrow cartilage results in normal AC in either structure or function.

This article summarizes the current techniques and how these techniques may evolve and presents some of the emerging techniques that are not yet in clinical use.

ADVANCES IN CURRENT RESTORATIVE THERAPIES

Although it is appealing to look to novel techniques to advance the science of cartilage repair, it is more likely that incremental advances in current techniques hold the most promise in the near future. The goal of re-establishing the native structure and function of native hyaline AC will take a biologic approach. The treatment of AC lesions is evolving from native tissue transplantation to engineering enhanced tissue, including cell- or gene-based therapy with 3D biodegradable scaffolds and growth factors (**Table 1**).[1–39]

Abrasion arthroplasty was one of the early techniques for surgical cartilage repair. The goal was to remove damaged cartilage and promote a healing response that would provide blood elements that would provide stable fibrocartilage for improved joint function.

Microfracture popularized in 1977 by Steadman and coworkers has been the more recent benchmark for cartilage repair from biologic tissue restorative techniques for pure cartilage defects. Steadman had good results for lesions less than 2.5 cm^2 in young patients.[3] This technique results in fibrocartilage as the repair tissue. As the science of cartilage repair advances, microfracture alone will likely see an increasingly limited role. It will very likely be that it will be used in combination with various growth factor and scaffold options.

Cartilage transplantation techniques were popularized to use hyaline cartilage in place of damaged AC. The use of osteochondral autograft transplantation (OAT) is typically used for lesions less than 4 cm^2 and fresh stored osteochondral allograft transplantation is used for lesions larger than 4 cm^2 (see **Table 1**).

The reported success of OAT procedures ranges from 50% to 80% as good to excellent. Some of the factors limiting success of this procedure include problems of cartilage thickness, graft orientation, graft contour, plug size versus defect size, use of donor versus defect shape mismatch, necessitating multiple round plugs and donor site problems. Currently this technique is best suited for defects less than 4 cm^2 primarily because of limited donor tissue. Changes in the technique that would likely improve the current technique include the following:

1. Allow different shaped donor plugs to accurately match the defect area;
2. Fill the donor site to minimize the defect in both the bone and cartilage;
3. Optimize the surface contour match between donor and recipient areas;
4. Optimize orientation of the cartilage surface for load-bearing and adjacent cartilage shear forces and to match adjacent native cartilage;
5. Assure plug fit so there is exact height match with surrounding surface;
6. Develop gap healing at graft-host boundary with fibrin glue or platelet-rich plasma;
7. Maintain existing chondrocyte viability through transfer (ie, using a no impact technique with graft insertion)

Table 1
Overview of regenerative therapy strategies for AC defects

	Advantages	Disadvantages
Currently existing treatment strategies		
Marrow-based stimulation: Microfracturing, drilling, 1980s	• One step procedure • To use bone marrow and progenitor cell • <2–4 cm^2 full-thickness cartilage	• Lack of differentiation into chondrocytes • Lack of cell containment • Lack of hyaline cartilage
Mosaicplasty or Osteochondral allografts and autografts transplantation: Cylindrical osteochondral plug or shell graft, 1992	• To directly use hyaline cartilage • <4 cm^2 for autograft; >4 cm^2 for allograft	• Donor site morbidity • Incomplete filling or matching the contour • High cost • Two-step procedures for allograft
Autologous Chondrocyte Implantation (ACI):	• Optimal cell retention • Minimize donor morbidity • To protect chondrocytes • >2cm^2 lesions	• Periosteal hyperplasia may limit joint motion • Two-step procedures
1st generation: a periosteal flap or collagen bilayer, 1994	• Create a reservoir by suture • 80%–90% good to excellent results	• Cell leakage • Prolonged postop activity restriction • Open procedure
2nd generation: bio-absorbable scaffolds or matrices (matrix autologous chondrocyte implantation), 2005	• Better secured scaffolds • Culture of chondrocytes on scaffolds with fibrin glue • Quicker and easier for arthroscopy	• Fewer cells • Two-step procedures • No long-term outcome
3rd generation: tissue engineered cell graft in 3D scaffold, 2005	• Well-simulated MSCs and progenitor cells in 3D scaffold • Hyaline cartilage-like tissue • Better in vivo regeneration	• No long-term outcome
Emerging treatment strategies		
Gene therapy	• A variety of sequences coding for humoral factors • Delivery of complementary DNA (cDNA) to growth factors and signal molecule (ie, adenoviral vectors, etc) • Ex vivo or in vivo inhibiting catabolic activity and inducing anabolic activity • See above at 3rd generation of ACI	• Experimental • Potential risk of viral introduction • See above at 3rd generation of ACI
Platelet-rich plasma or iliac crest bone marrow concentrate, 2006	• Inexpensive • Directly provide PDGF, TGF-β, FGF-2, and other mitogenic factors to a focal defect • Promote MSCs proliferation and chondrogenesis • Producing hyaline-like tissue	• Mainly animal experiments • One study showed poor clinical outcomes in 2-year follow-up

Data from Refs.[1–39]

Osteochondral allografting has become more popular over the last 20 years because of its ability to replace larger cartilage defects with a supportive subchondral and cancellous bony element. Here tissue quantity is not an issue as it is in OATs. Therefore, it is typically used for osteochondral defects larger than 4 cm^2 or when host donor tissue is not available or contraindicated. Problems associated with fresh osteochondral allografting include limited tissue availability (timing issue), requiring a separate procedure for insertion, limited chondrocyte viability, possible disease transmission, and tissue incorporation.

Developments that would significantly improve allografting results include the following:

1. Increase chondrocyte viability at time of grafting by reducing the wait times for early transplantation or improve chondrocyte preservation to prolong the window for transplantation;
2. Lower the small risk of disease transmission;
3. Improve the fit of shell grafts (for irregular or non–circular-shaped defects);
4. Improve contour and orientation.

Autologous chondrocyte implantation (ACI) is a cell-based treatment modality for full-thickness cartilage defects that has been used to repair AC defects since 1987 with good success.

It uses autologous chondrocytes transplanted into a defect with a periosteal patch or synthetic bilayer membrane cover in a 2-stage surgical technique. The harvested chondrocytes are grown in cell culture to a predetermined number and a confirmed viability level. The chondrocytes are then implanted using an open arthrotomy and implanted into the defect under the patch. In this technique there is no extracellular matrix or structural framework. It is up to the implanted complex along with the host factors to build the entire extracellular matrix so essential for the function and durability of native AC, which is a tall task for differentiated chondrocytes (see **Table 1**). Developments that could significantly improve the desired outcome of this technique include the following:

1. Selective chondrocyte implantation (also stem cells), improved membranes, and scaffolds;
2. Improved chondrocyte numbers, viability, perichondrium, biomembrane, and scaffold growth factors;
3. Improvements in cell viability, more rapid prerelease laboratory screening, tissue availability.

PROMISING CARTILAGE TISSUE ENGINEERING: SCAFFOLDS, GROWTH FACTORS, STEM CELL THERAPY

A cell-based approach to cartilage repair will likely require additions of both scaffold and growth factors. Scaffolds can be either collagen- or synthetic-based. Collagen is the major component of the physiologic and the extracellular cartilage matrix. Collagen provides most of the biomechanical properties essential for the mechanical function of cartilage, but also acts as a vehicle (scaffold) for cells. It also facilitates growth factor and cytokine transport into the cartilage lesions,[40] where cartilage repair, including fibrous tissue, fibrocartilage, or hyaline-cartilage-like tissue is initiated. It is a challenge to deliver either well-differentiated chondrocytes or mesenchymal stem and precursor cells (derived from bone marrow, periosteum, perichondrium, synovial tissue, adiposal or fibrous tissue) to the isolated cartilage defect. Investigations into the best therapeutic modality that offers a durable collagen scaffold with fewer side effects are ongoing.[41–43] The long-term outcome of implanted chondrocytes is still unknown. New technologies for cell delivery and a retention mechanism will need to be developed as a part of future therapeutic strategies (**Table 2**).

Collagen is not the only option for scaffolds for chondrocyte. Other (synthetic) types of scaffolds have been developed and their in vivo findings and performance are listed in **Table 3**.[68–91] Throughout in vivo and in vitro studies, chitosan-based material scaffolds are one of the most promising biopolymers in the regeneration therapy for AC defects.[69] Overall, the principles of functional scaffolds include the following:

1. Biocompatibility to alleviate inflammatory and immunologic response;
2. Appropriate 3D structure with retention of chondrocytes and sufficient porosity to allow ingrowth;
3. Ability to anchor and stabilize the cells on the lesion;

Table 2
Advantages and disadvantages for a group of collagen matrices as tools leading to the cartilage repair

Collagen Matrices	Advantages	Disadvantages
Cell-based:		
Collagen type I matrices	• Common: stabilize implants and differentiate cell • More fibroblastic cell growth • Better differentiation of MSC into chondrocyte phenotype	• Common: contraction • Less chondrocytic cells • Less glycosaminoglycans
Collagen type II matrices	• Common: stabilize implants and differentiate cell • More chondrocytic cell growth • More glycosaminoglycans • Increase type II accumulation in agarose and polylactic acid fleeces in vitro culture medium	• Common: contraction • Less fibroblastic cells
Cross-linking of collagen-glycosaminoglycan matrices: • Chondroitin sulfate with collagen type I • Carbodiimide with collagen type II	• Improved stiffness • Best promotion of chondrocyte growth • Stabilize matrices	• Need to investigate biocompatibility
Growth factors–based:		
• Biodegradable scaffolds with growth factors • Biodegradable microparticles or nanoparticles scaffolds with growth factors • Gene-activated matrix (BMP, IGF, TGF, bFGF)	• Increase metabolism of cells • Better regulate differentiation of cells • Efficiently induce a regenerative cascade • Entrap gene expression	• Experimental models • Also stimulate periosteal cells leading to chondrophyte • Do not deliver larger molecules

Data from Refs.[40,44–67]

Table 3
A brief of advantages and disadvantages for other major scaffolds important in cartilage repair

Scaffold	Advantages	Disadvantages
Natural proteic scaffolds: Collagen, gelatin, fibrin		
Fibrins	• Improved cartilage histology but still abnormal • Carries growth factor	• Poor mechanical properties • May evoke immune response • Lack of host cell ingrowth
Polysaccharidic scaffolds: Agarose, alginate, cellulose, chitosan, hyaluronic acid		
Agarose, Alginate	• Distribute cells evenly • Injectable • Good cartilage histology	• Poor mechanical properties • Less bioabsorbable • May evoke giant cell-like reaction • Weak cell adherence
Chitosan	• Excellent biocompatibility • Antibacterial nature • Ability to be molded with porosity • Good cell ingrowth and osteoconduction • Favorable gelling nature to deliver DNA, etc, molecules and pharmaceutical agents	• Questionable mechanical property
Hyaluronic acid	• Biocompatible • Integration with host	• May induce chondrolysis • Cartilage is thinner
Synthetic scaffolds: Carbon fiber, Calcium phosphate, polyesther urethane, polyglycolic acid, polylactic acid		
Polylactic acid	• Good cell containment • Integrates well with host together with BMP-2	• Induce variable bone growth • Poor quality of cartilage ingredient

Data from Refs.[68–91]

4. Biodegradability to enable cell differentiation and release of growth factors;
5. Adequate mechanical integrity.[68–91]

Several humoral factors play a significant role in the AC repair and induced regeneration. Those humoral factors have bioactive functions and may act indirectly through membrane receptors, signal pathways, or directly on the cartilage elements.[92] These factors are characterized by either anabolic effects or catabolic behaviors.[93] Their anabolic actions include an increase of matrix synthesis, promotion of chondrocyte differentiation, and improvement of cell migration. The catabolic actions are predominately responsible for the cartilage degeneration and cell necrosis. Those molecules mediate the metabolic cascade of chondrocyte development and homeostasis in the process of AC regeneration (**Table 4**). The use of multiple growth factors in the stimulation of cartilage regeneration may enhance cell differentiation or improve the modulation of terminal chondrogenesis.

Cell types that can be used for cartilage repair include differentiated chondrocytes like those used in autologous chondrocyte implantation procedures or nondifferentiated stem cells. Human stem cells are derived or obtained from adult (mature) or embryonic tissue. Embryonic stem cells are pluripotent cells derived from the blastocyst, whereas the adult stem cell has been found in most tissues in adults as well as in children and adolescents. Adult mesenchymal stem cells (MSCs) are involved in tissue homeostasis, remodeling, and regeneration and are replaced by mature cells during

Table 4
Function of major humoral factors in cartilage repair

Humoral Factors	Functions
Cartilaginous anabolic factors	
Transforming growth factor-β (TGF-β)	• Inducer of chondrogenesis of MSC • Stimulator of cartilage matrix expression and synthesis (type II collagen and aggrecan) • Inhibitor of osteogenic and adipogenic differentiation
BMPs-2, -5, -7	• Induce chondrogenic differentiation of MSC • Switch from immature collagen type II A to mature type II B
Insulin and insulin like growth factor 1(IGF-1)	• Control glucose metabolism in chondrocytes • Promote chondrocyte differentiation and stabilize cell phenotype
Fibroblast growth factors (FGFs)	• Promote chondrocyte proliferation and MSC differentiation, activation, and maintenance
Platelet-derived growth factor (PDGF)	• Mitogenic and chemotactic factor for chondrocyte and MSC • Promote heterotopic cartilage formation
Transcription factors (Sox 9)	• Regulator of chondrogenic differentiation • Drive the production of collagen type II • Increase expression of extracellular matrix (aggrecan)
Cartilaginous catabolic factors	
Interleukin-1	• Activation of catabolic pathway, including oxygen, PG, protease in initiation, and progression of degenerative AC
Tumor necrosis factor (TNF-α)	• Increase synthesis of catabolic enzymes

Data from Refs.[92–95]

the regenerative process.[96] Clinical application of adult stem cells has been widely reported by the use of bone marrow for MSCs. Not only can the adult MSCs be isolated from bone marrow but also can be generated from several other adult tissues, such as adipose, muscle, dermis, periosteum, synovial membrane and fluid, and AC.[97–112] MSCs are considered as having potential capability of differentiating along chondrogenic, osteogenic, and adipogenic pathways for generating cartilage, bone, and soft and connective tissues.

EMERGING TECHNOLOGIES FOR IMPROVING REGENERATIVE THERAPIES

Combining these evolving techniques using scaffold matrix populated with chondrogenic stem cells, augmented with appropriate growth factors, is no doubt the future of all cell-based cartilage repair strategies. Various externally applied therapies may enhance cartilage healing or regeneration. One such therapy is extracorporeal shock wave (ESW). Extracorporeal-generated shock waves were first introduced as a treatment of pulverizing kidney and ureteral stones in the 1980s. The longitudinal acoustic wave produced with ESW travels with the speed of ultrasound and creates a transient pressure wave that propagates rapidly in tissue. It can disintegrate kidney stones but can a have a more subtle effect on soft tissues through stimulation of various cellular and extracellular processes.[43]

These effects of ESW on cartilage include induction of angiogenesis, recruitment of progenitor cells, and reduction of cartilage damage. Vascular endothelial growth factor (VEGF) is a chemical signal produced by cells, which stimulates endothelial cell proliferation, promotes neovascularization, and increases vascular permeability. After the use of shockwave therapy to the necrotic femoral heads of rabbits, VEGF mRNA expression was significantly up-regulated. The up-regulation of VEGF may play a role in improving blood supply to the osteochondral lesions and facilitating healing.[42] ESW was able to diminish chondrocyte inflammation and apoptosis while increasing cell viability. The mechanism of ESW may relate to the restoration of mitochondrial function and regulation of nitric oxide (NO) and cytokine release. Similar studies in the rabbit model with osteoarthritis (OA) and rat model with OA showed a significant decrease in the cartilage degradation, an increase in chondrocyte activity, and a reduction of the NO.[113,114] Both human AC and human OA models were also investigated following the use of ESW, displaying a down-regulation of the intracellular levels of TNF-α and interleukin-10 in chondrocytes, reducing overall joint inflammation.[115]

ESW has been used to treat various tendinopathies, such as calcific tendinitis of the shoulder, lateral elbow epicondylitis, and plantar fasciitis. Its role is expanding to treatment of orthopedic conditions, including osteochondral defects, femoral head necrosis, delayed unions, and nonunions of fractures.[116–126] It is thought that using ESW treatment on AC stimulates the healing process or reactivates the growth process in cartilage, bone, tendon, and surrounding tissues, occurring when microdisruption is induced into both avascular and minimally vascular tissue stimulating revascularization. This revascularization then proceeds to recruit growth factors and even possibly stem cells that are necessary for normal healing.[117,126] Lyon and colleagues[127] used ESW applied to a 4-mm-diameter osteochondral plug on the medial femoral condyle in a rabbit model with a single application of 4000 impulses. The histologic results found that there was mature bone formation, better healing, and improved density of the cartilage on the treated side as compared with the control side, demonstrating its therapeutic value in accelerating the healing rate while improving cartilage and subchondral bone quality. Despite the fact there are variable findings directly related to the healing of the subchondral bone structure, the increases in osteocalcin, collagen I and II, and proteoglycan aggrecan strongly support the use of ESW in subchondral bone remodeling.[128,129]

As a result of morphologic, histologic, immunohistochemical, and biologic investigation on the cartilage, bone, and soft tissue, it is postulated that ESW may alter the process of angiogenic and osteogenic growth factors, endothelial NO synthase, VEGF, bone morphogenetic proteins (BMP-2), and proliferating cell nuclear antigen, which may profoundly improve AC and subchondral bone remodeling and enhance the cartilage repair.[130] This alteration makes ESW a possible alternative or at least augmentation of the various (in vivo or in vitro) cartilage restoration techniques. As an example, ESW could be used before the standard treatments of cartilage defects. A single-stage treatment on the bone marrow, mesenchymal stem cell, chondrocytes, minced cartilage, even on the autograft and allograft, could be a helpful adjunct (**Fig. 1**).

FUTURE DIRECTIONS OF THE TISSUE ENGINEERING THERAPY FOR AC DEFECTS

There are multiple questions yet to be answered to move the science of cartilage repair forward. These treatment strategies, such as bone marrow–based stimulation, OAT, ACI, and matrix autologous chondrocyte implantation, are capable of repairing

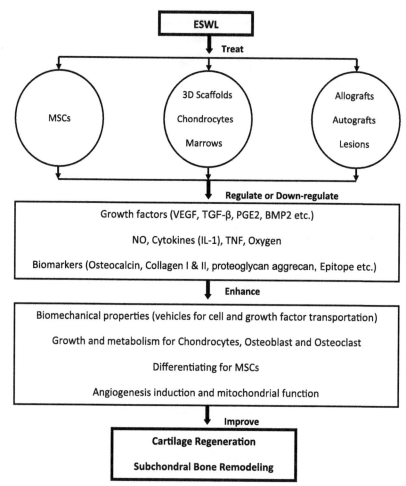

Fig. 1. Prospective and enhancement of the ESWL on the cartilage regeneration and bone remodeling in the AC defects.

and regenerating hyaline-like cartilage in the different qualities. There are no gold standards in treatment strategies currently identified in the regeneration of AC. Still lacking are the long-term clinical outcomes from multiple centers with level I evidence for MSCs and gene-based therapy. The biodegradable, biocompatible, and biomechanical characteristics of the matrix and growth factors in coupling with the MSC's differentiation and proliferation still remain unresolved. Converting experimental findings to clinical trials and clinical application will benefit patients with AC lesions (**Fig. 2**).

Another important aspect in the advancement of cartilage repair is the development of clear indications, contraindications, recommended techniques, and postoperative rehabilitation protocols. It is crucial that a specific technique be appropriately matched with the existing cartilage lesion and not used blindly no matter the circumstances of the lesion or the patient. Also needed is a better understanding of the difference between an acute traumatic cartilage defect in a normal joint and a cartilage defect in a pathologic joint. Joint pathologies can include degenerative arthritis, chronic synovitis, infection, mal-alignment, kissing lesions, and aging issues. Without resolution of

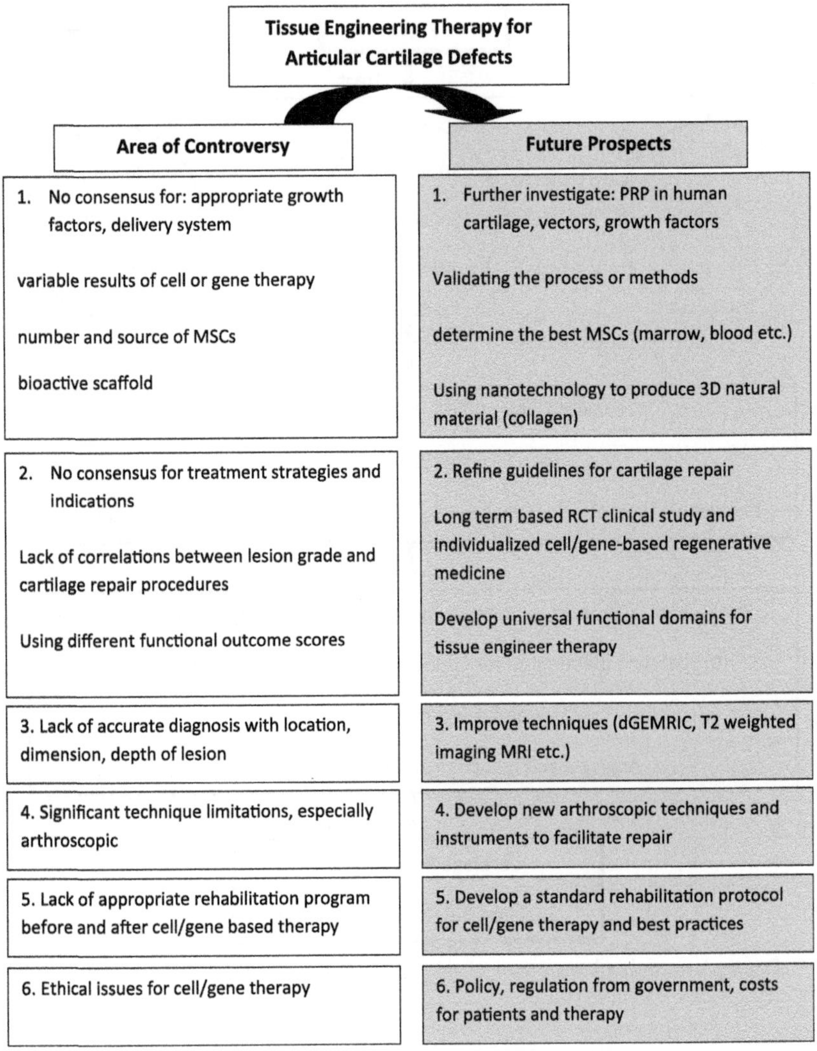

Tissue Engineering Therapy for Articular Cartilage Defects	
Area of Controversy	**Future Prospects**
1. No consensus for: appropriate growth factors, delivery system	1. Further investigate: PRP in human cartilage, vectors, growth factors
variable results of cell or gene therapy	Validating the process or methods
number and source of MSCs	determine the best MSCs (marrow, blood etc.)
bioactive scaffold	Using nanotechnology to produce 3D natural material (collagen)
2. No consensus for treatment strategies and indications	2. Refine guidelines for cartilage repair
Lack of correlations between lesion grade and cartilage repair procedures	Long term based RCT clinical study and individualized cell/gene-based regenerative medicine
Using different functional outcome scores	Develop universal functional domains for tissue engineer therapy
3. Lack of accurate diagnosis with location, dimension, depth of lesion	3. Improve techniques (dGEMRIC, T2 weighted imaging MRI etc.)
4. Significant technique limitations, especially arthroscopic	4. Develop new arthroscopic techniques and instruments to facilitate repair
5. Lack of appropriate rehabilitation program before and after cell/gene based therapy	5. Develop a standard rehabilitation protocol for cell/gene therapy and best practices
6. Ethical issues for cell/gene therapy	6. Policy, regulation from government, costs for patients and therapy

Fig. 2. Controversy and future directions of tissue engineering therapy for AC defects.

joint pathologic abnormality, the use of cartilage repair techniques may be contraindicated or at least have very limited benefit. Therefore, development of best practice recommendations could greatly improve outcomes. Also, development of centers of excellence that understand and follow the advanced care plans could lead to significant improvements in outcomes even without significant scientific advancements (see **Fig. 2**).

The role of the US Food and Drug Administration (FDA) and government regulation is a mixed bag. FDA approval is necessary for widespread use of techniques in cartilage repair. Although the FDA is not the source of innovations or improvements, it should make more effort to promote the advancement of cartilage repair techniques. Legislative actions on stem cells and clinical adoption of scientific advancement should direct and strengthen the pace of new regenerative strategies (see **Fig. 2**).

SUMMARY

The near future of cartilage repair will most likely involve refinement of current techniques along with incorporation of scientific advances in cartilage biology. With further development, the implantation of a scaffold imbedded with stem cells and cartilage growth factors will likely be scientifically achievable and it is to be hoped that it could be made clinically viable and cost-effective. Ongoing research into cartilage repair should offer single-stage surgical technique, which will replicate the structural characteristics of normal articular (hyaline) cartilage and incorporate onto bone.

REFERENCES

1. Gomoll AH. Microfracture and augments. J Knee Surg 2012;25(1):9–15.
2. Steadman JR, Rodkey WG, Rodrigo JJ. Microfracture: surgical technique and rehabilitation to treat chondral defects. Clin Orthop Relat Res 2001;(Suppl 391):S362–9.
3. Steadman JR, Miller BS, Karas SG, et al. The microfracture technique in the treatment of full thickness chondral lesions of the knee in National Football League players. J Knee Surg 2003;16(2):83–6.
4. Hurst JM, Steadman JR, O'Brien L, et al. Rehabilitation following microfracture for chondral injury in the knee. Clin Sports Med 2010;29(2):257–65, viii.
5. McCoy B, Miniaci A. Osteochondral autograft transplantation/mosaicplasty. J Knee Surg 2012;25(2):99–108.
6. Hangody L, Fules P. Autologous osteochondral mosaicplasty for the treatment of full-thickness defects of weight-bearing joints: ten years of experimental and clinical experience. J Bone Joint Surg Am 2003;85-A(Suppl 2):25–32.
7. Bentley G, Biant LC, Carrington RW, et al. A prospective, randomised comparison of autologous chondrocyte implantation versus mosaicplasty for osteochondral defects in the knee. J Bone Joint Surg Br 2003;85(2):223–30.
8. Bentley G, Biant LC, Vijayan S, et al. Minimum ten-year results of a prospective randomised study of autologous chondrocyte implantation versus mosaicplasty for symptomatic articular cartilage lesions of the knee. J Bone Joint Surg Br 2012;94(4):504–9.
9. Dozin B, Malpeli M, Cancedda R, et al. Comparative evaluation of autologous chondrocyte implantation and mosaicplasty: a multicentered randomized clinical trial. Clin J Sport Med 2005;15(4):220–6.
10. Peterson L, Minas T, Brittberg M, et al. Treatment of osteochondritis dissecans of the knee with autologous chondrocyte transplantation: results at two to ten years. J Bone Joint Surg Am 2003;85-A(Suppl 2):17–24.
11. Tuan RS. A second-generation autologous chondrocyte implantation approach to the treatment of focal articular cartilage defects. Arthritis Res Ther 2007; 9(5):109.
12. Behrens P, Bitter T, Kurz B, et al. Matrix-associated autologous chondrocyte transplantation/implantation (MACT/MACI) – 5-year follow-up. Knee 2006; 13(3):194–202.
13. Minas T, Gomoll AH, Solhpour S, et al. Autologous chondrocyte implantation for joint preservation in patients with early osteoarthritis. Clin Orthop Relat Res 2010;468(1):147–57.
14. Rosenberger RE, Gomoll AH, Bryant T, et al. Repair of large chondral defects of the knee with autologous chondrocyte implantation in patients 45 years or older. Am J Sports Med 2008;36(12):2336–44.

15. Bartlett W, Skinner JA, Gooding CR, et al. Autologous chondrocyte implantation versus matrix-induced autologous chondrocyte implantation for osteochondral defects of the knee: a prospective, randomised study. J Bone Joint Surg Br 2005;87(5):640–5.

16. Dickinson SC, Sims TJ, Pittarello L, et al. Quantitative outcome measures of cartilage repair in patients treated by tissue engineering. Tissue Eng 2005; 11(1–2):277–87.

17. Saris DB, Vanlauwe J, Victor J, et al. Characterized chondrocyte implantation results in better structural repair when treating symptomatic cartilage defects of the knee in a randomized controlled trial versus microfracture. Am J Sports Med 2008;36(2):235–46.

18. Aroen A, Løken S, Heir S, et al. Articular cartilage lesions in 993 consecutive knee arthroscopies. Am J Sports Med 2004;32(1):211–5.

19. Flanigan DC, Harris JD, Trinh TQ, et al. Prevalence of chondral defects in athletes' knees: a systematic review. Med Sci Sports Exerc 2010;42(10):1795–801.

20. Heir S, Nerhus TK, Røtterud JH, et al. Focal cartilage defects in the knee impair quality of life as much as severe osteoarthritis: a comparison of knee injury and osteoarthritis outcome score in 4 patient categories scheduled for knee surgery. Am J Sports Med 2010;38(2):231–7.

21. Lane JG, Massie JB, Ball ST, et al. Follow-up of osteochondral plug transfers in a goat model: a 6-month study. Am J Sports Med 2004;32:1440–50.

22. Rose T, Craatz S, Hepp P, et al. The autologous osteochondral transplantation of the knee: clinical results, radiographic findings and histological aspects. Arch Orthop Trauma Surg 2005;125:628–37.

23. Beaver RJ, Mahomed M, Backstein D, et al. Fresh osteochondral allografts for post-traumatic defects in the knee. A survivorship analysis. J Bone Joint Surg Br 1992;74:105–10.

24. Minas T. Autologous chondrocyte implantation for focal chondral defects of the knee. Clin Orthop Relat Res 2001;(Suppl 391):S349–61.

25. Kreuz PC, Steinwachs M, Erggelet C, et al. Classification of graft hypertrophy after autologous chondrocyte implantation of full-thickness chondral defects in the knee. Osteoarthritis Cartilage 2007;15:1339–47.

26. Micheli LJ, Browne JE, Erggelet C, et al. Autologous chondrocyte implantation of the knee: multicenter experience and minimum 3-year follow-up. Clin J Sport Med 2001;11:223–8.

27. Marlovits S, Striessnig G, Kutscha-Lissberg F, et al. Early postoperative adherence of matrix-induced autologous chondrocyte implantation for the treatment of full-thickness cartilage defects of the femoral condyle. Knee Surg Sports Traumatol Arthrosc 2005;13:451–7.

28. Jones CW, Willers C, Keogh A, et al. Matrix-induced autologous chondrocyte implantation in sheep: objective assessments including confocal arthroscopy. J Orthop Res 2008;26:292–303.

29. Torzilli PA, Bhargava M, Park S, et al. Mechanical load inhibits IL-1 induced matrix degradation in articular cartilage. Osteoarthritis Cartilage 2010;18(1): 97–105.

30. Tanimoto K, Kitamura R, Tanne Y, et al. Modulation of hyaluronan catabolism in chondrocytes by mechanical stimuli. J Biomed Mater Res A 2010;93(1):373–80.

31. Ryan JA, Eisner EA, DuRaine G, et al. Mechanical compression of articular cartilage induces chondrocyte proliferation and inhibits proteoglycan synthesis by activation of the ERK pathway: implications for tissue engineering and regenerative medicine. J Tissue Eng Regen Med 2009;3:107–16.

32. Mishra A, Tummala P, King A, et al. Buffered platelet-rich plasma enhances mesenchymal stem cell proliferation and chondrogenic differentiation. Tissue Eng Part C Methods 2009;15:431–5.
33. Akeda K, An HS, Okuma M, et al. Platelet-rich plasma stimulates porcine articular chondrocyte proliferation and matrix biosynthesis. Osteoarthritis Cartilage 2006;14:1272–80.
34. Everts PA, Knape JT, Weibrich G, et al. Platelet-rich plasma and platelet gel: a review. J Extra Corpor Technol 2006;38:174–87.
35. Ishida K, Kuroda R, Miwa M, et al. The regenerative effects of platelet-rich plasma on meniscal cells in vitro and its in vivo application with biodegradable gelatin hydrogel. Tissue Eng 2007;13:1103–12.
36. Wu W, Chen F, Liu Y, et al. Autologous injectable tissue-engineered cartilage by using platelet-rich plasma: experimental study in a rabbit model. J Oral Maxillofac Surg 2007;65:1951–7.
37. Brehm W, Aklin B, Yamashita T, et al. Repair of superficial osteochondral defects with an autologous scaffold-free cartilage construct in a caprine model: implantation method and short-term results. Osteoarthritis Cartilage 2006;14:1214–26.
38. Kon E, Buda R, Filardo G, et al. Platelet-rich plasma: intra-articular knee injections produced favorable results on degenerative cartilage lesions. Knee Surg Sports Traumatol Arthrosc 2010;18(4):472–9.
39. Filardo G, Kon E, Buda R, et al. Platelet-rich plasma intra-articular knee injections for the treatment of degenerative cartilage lesions and osteoarthritis. Knee Surg Sports Traumatol Arthrosc 2011;19(4):528–35.
40. Aigner T, Stove J. Collagens-major component of the physiological cartilage matrix, major target of cartilage degeneration, major tool in cartilage repair. Adv Drug Deliv Rev 2003;55:1569–93.
41. Gelse K, Jiang QJ, Aigner T, et al. Fibroblast-mediated delivery of growth factor complementary DNA into mouse joints induces chondrogenesis but avoids the disadvantages of direct viral gene transfer. Arthritis Rheum 2011;44:1943–53.
42. Maier M, Averbeck B, Milz S, et al. Substance P and prostaglandin E_2 release after shock wave application to the rabbit femur. Clin Orthop Relat Res 2003;406:237–45.
43. Ogden J, Toth A, Schultheiss R. Principles of shock wave therapy. Clin Orthop Relat Res 2001;387:8–17.
44. Kimura T, Yasui N, Ohsawa S, et al. Chondrocytes embedded in collagen gels maintain cartilage phenotype during long-term cultures. Clin Orthop 1984;186:231–9.
45. Ehlers EM, Fuss M, Rohwedel J, et al. Development of a biocomposite to fill out articular cartilage lesions. Light, scanning and transmission electron microscopy of sheep chondrocytes cultured on a collagen I/III sponge. Anat Anz 1999;181:513–8.
46. Katsube K, Ochi M, Uchio Y, et al. Repair of articular cartilage defects with cultured chondrocytes in Atelocollagen gel. Comparison with cultured chondrocytes in suspension. Arch Orthop Trauma Surg 2000;120:121–7.
47. Sams AE, Minor RR, Wootton JA, et al. Local and remote matrix responses to chondrocyte-laden collagen scaffold implantation in extensive articular cartilage defects. Osteoarthritis Cartilage 1995;3:61–70.
48. Lee CR, Breinan HA, Nehrer S, et al. Articular cartilage chondrocytes in type I and type II collagen-GAG matrices exhibit contractile behavior in vitro. Tissue Eng 2000;6:555–65.

49. Nehrer S, Breinan HA, Ramappa A, et al. Matrix collagen type and pore size influence behaviour of seeded canine chondrocytes. Biomaterials 1997;18: 769–76.

50. Lee CR, Grodzinsky AJ, Spector M. The effects of crosslinking of collagen –glycosaminoglycan scaffolds on compressive stiffness, chondrocyte-mediated contraction, proliferation and biosynthesis. Biomaterials 2001;22:3145–54.

51. D'Lima DD, Hashimoto S, Chen PC, et al. Human chondrocyte apoptosis in response to mechanical injury. Osteoarthritis Cartilage 2001;9:712–9.

52. Tsai CL, Hsu SH, Cheng WL. Effect of different solvents and crosslinkers on cytocompatibility of Type II collagen scaffolds for chondrocyte seeding. Artif Organs 2002;26:18–26.

53. Van Susante JL, Pieper J, Buma P, et al. Linkage of chondroitin-sulfate to type I collagen scaffolds stimulates the bioactivity of seeded chondrocytes in vitro. Biomaterials 2001;22:2359–69.

54. Van Wachem PB, Van Luyn MJ, OldeDamink LH, et al. Biocompatibility and tissue regenerating capacity of crosslinked dermal sheep collagen. J Biomed Mater Res 1994;28:353–63.

55. Pieper JS, Oosterhof A, Dijkstra PJ, et al. Preparation and characterization of porous crosslinked collagenous matrices containing bioavailable chondroitin sulphate. Biomaterials 1999;20:847–58.

56. Freed LE, Vunjak-Novakovic G, Langer R. Cultivation of cell-polymer cartilage implants in bioreactors. J Cell Biochem 1999;51(3):257–64.

57. Gugala Z, Gogolewski S. In vitro growth and activity of primary chondrocytes on a resorbable polylactide three-dimensional scaffold. J Biomed Mater Res 2000; 49:183–91.

58. Lu L, Stamatas GN, Mikos AG. Controlled release of transforming growth factor beta1 from biodegradable polymer microparticles. J Biomed Mater Res 2000; 50:440–51.

59. Peter SJ, Lu L, Kim DJ, et al. Effects of transforming growth factor beta1 released from biodegradable polymer microparticles on marrow stromal osteoblasts cultured on poly(propylene fumarate) substrates. J Biomed Mater Res 2000;50:452–62.

60. Bonadio J, Smiley E, Patil P, et al. Localized, direct plasmid gene delivery in vivo: prolonged therapy results in reproducible tissue regeneration. Nat Med 1999;5:753–9.

61. Bonadio J. Tissue engineering via local gene delivery. J Mol Med 2000;78: 303–11.

62. Friedlaender GE, Perry CR, Cole JD, et al. Osteogenic protein-1 (bone morphogenetic protein-7) in the treatment of tibial nonunions. J Bone Joint Surg Am 2001;83-A(Suppl 1):S151–8.

63. Trippel SB. Growth factor actions on articular cartilage. J Rheumatol 1995;22: 129–32.

64. Nixon AJ, Fortier LA, Williams J, et al. Enhanced repair of extensive articular cartilage defects by insulin-like growth factor-I-laden fibrin composites. J Orthop Res 1999;17:475–87.

65. Domowicz M, Krueger RC, Li H, et al. The nanomelic mutation in the aggrecan gene is expressed in chick chondrocytes and neurons. Int J Dev Neurosci 1996; 14:191–201.

66. Fujimoto E, Ochi M, Kato Y, et al. Beneficial effect of fibroblast growth factor on the repair of full thickness defects in rabbit articular cartilage. Arch Orthop Trauma Surg 1999;119:139–45.

67. Otsuka Y, Mizuta H, Takagi K, et al. Requirement of fibroblast growth factor signaling for regeneration of epiphyseal morphology in rabbit full thickness defects of articular cartilage. Dev Growth Differ 1997;39:143–56.
68. Frenkel S, Cesare PE. Scaffolds for articular repair. Ann Biomed Eng 2004;32(1): 26–34.
69. Martino AD, Sittinger M, Risbud M. Chitosan: a versatile biopolymer for orthopaedic tissue-engineering. Biomaterials 2005;26:5983–90.
70. Brittberg M, Sjogren-Jansson E, Lindahl A, et al. Influence of fibrin sealant (Tisseel) on osteochondral defect repair in the rabbit knee. Biomaterials 1997; 18:235–42.
71. Hendrickson DA, Nixon AJ, Grande DA, et al. Chondrocyte-fibrin matrix transplants for resurfacing extensive articular cartilage defects. J Orthop Res 1994;12:485–96.
72. Nixon AJ, Saxer R, Brower-Toland B. Exogenous insulin-like growth factor-I stimulates an autoinductive IGF-I autocrine/paracrine response in chondrocytes. J Orthop Res 2001;19:26–32.
73. Van Susante JL, Buma P, Schuman L, et al. Resurfacing potential of heterologous chondrocytes suspended in fibrin glue in large full-thickness defects of femoral articular cartilage: an experimental study in the goat. Biomaterials 1999;20:1167–75.
74. Dausse Y, Grossin L, Miralles G, et al. Cartilage repair using new polysaccharidic biomaterials: macroscopic, histological and biochemical approaches in a rat model of cartilage defect. Osteoarthritis Cartilage 2003;11:16–28.
75. Diduch DR, Jordan L, Mierisch C, et al. Marrow stromal cells embedded in alginate for repair of osteochondral defects. Arthroscopy 2000;16:571–7.
76. Marijnissen WJ, Van Osch G, Aigner G, et al. Tissue-engineered cartilage using serially passaged articular chondrocytes. Chondrocytes in alginate, combined in vivo with a synthetic (E210) or biologic biodegradable carrier (DBM). Biomaterials 2000;21:571–80.
77. Weisser J, Rahfoth B, Timmermann A, et al. Role of growth factors in rabbit articular cartilage repair by chondrocytes in agarose. Osteoarthritis Cartilage 2001; 9A:S48–54.
78. Butnariu-Ephrat M, Robinson D, Mendes D, et al. Resurfacing of goat articular cartilage by chondrocytes derived from bone marrow. Clin Orthop 1996;330: 234–43.
79. Gao J, Dennis J, Solchaga L, et al. Repair of osteochondral defect with tissue-engineered two-phase composite material of injectable calcium phosphate and hyaluronan sponge. Tissue Eng 2002;8:827–37.
80. Knudson W, Casey B, Nishida Y, et al. Hyaluronan oligosaccharides perturb cartilage matrix homeostasis and induce chondrocytic chondrolysis. Arthritis Rheum 2000;43:1165–74.
81. Marcacci M, Zaffagnini S, Kon E, et al. Arthroscopic autologous chondrocyte transplantation: technical note. Knee Surg Sports Traumatol Arthrosc 2002;10: 154–9.
82. Chu CR, Dounchis J, Yoshioka M, et al. Osteochondral repair using perichondrial cells. A 1-year study in rabbits. Clin Orthop 1997;340:220–9.
83. Dounchis JS, Bae W, Chen A, et al. Cartilage repair with autogenic perichondrium cell and polylactic acid grafts. Clin Orthop 2000;377:248–64.
84. Frenkel SR, Bradica G, Brekke JH, et al. Regeneration of articular cartilage-evaluation of osteochondral defect repair in the rabbit using multiphasic implants. Osteoarthritis Cartilage 2005;13(9):798–807.

85. Giurea A, Klein T, Chen A, et al. Adhesion of perichondrial cells to a polylactic acid scaffold. J Orthop Res 2003;21:584–9.

86. Clouet J, Vinatier C, Merceron C, et al. Therapeutic strategies for the effective management of OA and cartilage defects: from osteoarthritis treatment to future regenerative therapies for cartilage. Drug Discov Today 2009;14(19–20): 913–25.

87. Nesic D, Whiteside R, Brittberg M, et al. Cartilage tissue engineering for degenerative joint disease. Adv Drug Deliv Rev 2006;58:300–22.

88. Elisseeff J. Injectable cartilage tissue engineering. Expert Opin Biol Ther 2004;4: 1849–59.

89. Drury JL, Mooney DJ. Hydrogels for tissue engineering: scaffold design variables and applications. Biomaterials 2003;24:4337–51.

90. Sontjens SH, Nettles DL, Carnahan MA, et al. Biodendrimer-based hydrogel scaffolds for cartilage tissue repair. Biomacromolecules 2006;7:310–6.

91. Vinatier C, Magne D, Moreau A, et al. Engineering cartilage with human nasal chondrocytes and a silanized hydroxypropyl methylcellulose hydrogel. J Biomed Mater Res 2007;A80:66–74.

92. Gaissmaier C, Koh JL, Weise K. Growth and differentiation factors for cartilage healing and repair. Injury 2008;39(Suppl 1):S88–96.

93. Freyria AM, Mallein-Gerin F. Chondrocytes or adult stem cells for cartilage repair: the indisputable role of growth factors. Injury 2012;43:259–65.

94. Kerker J, Leo AL, Sgaglione NA. Cartilage repair: synthetics and scaffolds. Sports Med Arthrosc 2008;16(4):208–16.

95. de Crombrugghe B, Lefebvre V, Behringer RR, et al. Transcriptional mechanisms of chondrocyte differentiation. Matrix Biol 2000;19:389–94.

96. De Bari C, Dell'Accio F. Mesenchymal stem cells in rheumatology: a regenerative approach to joint repair. Clin Sci (Lond) 2007;113:339–48.

97. Friedenstein AJ, Chailakhjan RK, Lalykina KS. The development of fibroblast colonies in monolayer cultures of guinea-pig bone marrow and spleen cells. Cell Tissue Kinet 1970;3:393–403.

98. Pittenger MF, Mackay AM, Beck SC, et al. Multilineage potential of adult human mesenchymal stem cells. Science 1999;284:143–7.

99. Caplan AI. Mesenchymal stem cells. J Orthop Res 1991;9:641–50.

100. Caplan AI, Bruder SP. Mesenchymal stem cells: building blocks for molecular medicine in the 21st century. Trends Mol Med 2001;7:259–64.

101. Prockop DJ. Marrow stromal cells as stem cells for nonhematopoietic tissues. Science 1997;276:71–4.

102. De Bari C, Dell'Accio F, Tylzanowski P, et al. Multipotent mesenchymal stem cells from adult human synovial membrane. Arthritis Rheum 2001;44:1928–42.

103. De Bari C, Dell'Accio F, Vandenabeele F, et al. Skeletal muscle repair by adult human mesenchymal stem cells from synovial membrane. J Cell Biol 2003; 160:909–18.

104. De Bari C, Dell'Accio F, Luyten FP. Failure of in vitro-differentiated mesenchymal stem cells from the synovial membrane to form ectopic stable cartilage in vivo. Arthritis Rheum 2004;50:142–50.

105. Jones EA, English A, Henshaw K, et al. Enumeration and phenotypic characterization of synovial fluid multipotential mesenchymal progenitor cells in inflammatory and degenerative arthritis. Arthritis Rheum 2004;50:817–27.

106. De Bari C, Dell'Accio F, Luyten FP. Human periosteum-derived cells maintain phenotypic stability and chondrogenic potential throughout expansion regardless of donor age. Arthritis Rheum 2001;44:85–95.

107. De Bari C, Dell'Accio F, Vanlauwe J, et al. Mesenchymal multipotency of adult human periosteal cells demonstrated by single cell lineage analysis. Arthritis Rheum 2006;54:1209–21.

108. Dell'Accio F, De Bari C, Luyten FP. Microenvironment and phenotypic stability specify tissue formation by human articular cartilage-derived cells in vivo. Exp Cell Res 2003;287:16–27.

109. Dowthwaite GP, Bishop JC, Redman SN, et al. The surface of articular cartilage contains a progenitor cell population. J Cell Sci 2004;117:889–97.

110. Barbero A, Ploegert S, Heberer M, et al. Plasticity of clonal populations of dedifferentiated adult human articular chondrocytes. Arthritis Rheum 2003;48: 1315–25.

111. Alsalameh S, Amin R, Gemba T, et al. Identification of mesenchymal progenitor cells in normal and osteoarthritic human articular cartilage. Arthritis Rheum 2004;50:1522–32.

112. Richardson SM, Hoyland JA, Mobasheri R, et al. Mesenchymal stem cells in regenerative medicine: opportunities and challenges for articular cartilage and intervertebral disc tissue engineering. J Cell Physiol 2009; 222:23–32.

113. Zhao Z, Ji HR, Jing RF, et al. Extracorporal shock-wave therapy reduces progression of the knee osteoarthritis in rabbits by reducing nitric oxide level and chondrocyte apoptosis. Arch Orthop Trauma Surg 2012;132:1547–53.

114. Wang CJ, Weng LH, Ko JY, et al. Extracorporeal shockwave therapy shows chondroprotective effects in osteoarthritic rat knee. Arch Orthop Trauma Surg 2011;131:1153–8.

115. Moretti B, Lannone F, Notarnicola A, et al. Extracorporeal shock waves downregulate the expression of interleukin-10 and tumor necrosis factor-alpha in osteoarthritic chondrocytes. BMC Musculoskelet Disord 2008;9:16.

116. Gerdesmeyer L, Wagenpfeil S, Haake M, et al. Extracorporeal shock wave therapy for the treatment of chronic calcifying tendonitis of the rotator cuff. JAMA 2003;290:2573–80.

117. Ogden JA, Alvarez RG, Levitt RL, et al. Electrohydraulic high-energy shockwave treatment for chronic plantar fasciitis. J Bone Joint Surg Am 2004;86-A: 2216–28.

118. Norman D, Reis D, Zinman C, et al. Vascular deprivation-induced necrosis of the femoral head of the rat. An experimental model of avascular osteonecrosis in the skeletally immature individual or Legg-Perthes disease. Int J Exp Pathol 1998; 79:173–9.

119. Ogden JA, Alvarez RG, Levitt R, et al. Shock wave therapy (orthotripsy) in musculoskeletal disorders. Clin Orthop Relat Res 2001;387:22–40.

120. Ludwig J, Lauber S, Lauber HS, et al. High-energy shock wave treatment of femoral head necrosis in adults. Clin Orthop Relat Res 2001;387:119–26.

121. Rompe JD, Kirkpatrick CJ, Kullmer K, et al. Dose-related effects of shock waves on rabbit tendo Achillis. A sonographic and histological study. J Bone Joint Surg Br 1998;80-B:546–52.

122. Sauer ST, Marymont JV, Mizel MS. What's new in foot and ankle surgery. J Bone Joint Surg Am 2004;86-A:878–86.

123. Thiel M. Application of shock waves in medicine. Clin Orthop Relat Res 2001; 387:18–21.

124. Vaterlein N, Lussenhop S, Hahn M, et al. The effect of extracorporeal shock waves on joint cartilage – an in vivo study in rabbits. Arch Orthop Trauma Surg 2000;120:403–6.

125. Wang CJ, Huang HY, Chen HH, et al. Effect of shock wave therapy on acute fractures of the tibia. Clin Orthop Relat Res 2001;387:112–8.
126. Wang CJ, Wang FS, Yang KD, et al. Shock wave therapy induces neovascularization at the tendon-bone junction. J Orthop Res 2003;21:984–9.
127. Lyon R, Liu XC, Kubin M, et al. Does extracorporeal shock wave therapy enhance healing of on OCD of the rabbit knee?: a pilot study. Clin Orthop Relat Res 2013;471(4):1159–65.
128. Kawcak CE, Frisbie DD, Mcilwraith W. Effects of extracorporal shock wave therapy and polysulfated glycosaminoglycan treatment on subchondral bone, serum biomarkers, and synovial fluid biomarkers in horses with induced osteoarthritis. Am J Vet Res 2011;72(6):772–9.
129. Wang CJ, Sun YC, Wong T, et al. Extracorporal shockwave therapy shows time-dependent chondroprotective effects in osteoarthritis of the knee in rats. J Surg Res 2012;178:196–205.
130. Lyon R, Liu XC, An JZ, et al. Extracorporeal pulse activation on the mitochondrial function and nitric oxide release in LPS-treated chondrocytes. 13th Annual Congress of the International Society for Medical Shockwave Treatment (ISMST). Chicago, June 24–26, 2010.

Physical Therapy Management of Patients with Osteochondritis Dissecans: A Comprehensive Review

Mark V. Paterno, PT, PhD, SCS, ATC[a,b,c,d,*],
Tricia R. Prokop, PT, MS, CSCS[e,f], Laura C. Schmitt, PT, PhD[a,b,g]

KEYWORDS

- Osteochondritis dissecans • Rehabilitation • Return to activity
- Non-operative management • Post-operative management

KEY POINTS

- Physical therapy management of osteochondritis dissecans can incorporate a full spectrum of conservative, nonoperative, and postoperative care.
- Rehabilitation interventions can vary based on factors such as the lesion characteristics, lesion location, articular cartilage involvement, skeletal maturity of the patient, presenting impairments at the time of evaluation, and concomitant injury.
- It is the responsibility of the rehabilitation professional to address all corresponding factors and mindfully advance the patient with a systematic and evidence-based progression to protect healing tissue and optimize outcome.

INTRODUCTION

Osteochondritis dissecans (OCD) refers to a lesion or injury of the subchondral bone, which may or may not involve the integrity of articular cartilage.[1–4] It has most recently been defined as a focal idiopathic alteration of subchondral bone with risk for

[a] Cincinnati Children's Hospital Medical Center, 3333 Burnet Avenue, MLC 10001, Cincinnati, OH 45229, USA; [b] Division of Sports Medicine, Cincinnati Children's Hospital Medical Center, 3333 Burnet Avenue, Cincinnati, OH 45229, USA; [c] Division of Occupational Therapy and Physical Therapy, Cincinnati Children's Hospital Medical Center, 3333 Burnet Avenue, Cincinnati, OH, USA; [d] Department of Pediatrics, College of Medicine, University of Cincinnati, Cincinnati, OH, USA; [e] Connecticut Children's Medical Center, Department of Physical Therapy, Division of Sports Medicine, Hartford, CT 06106, USA; [f] Department of Rehabilitation Sciences, College of Education, Nursing, and Health Professionals, University of Hartford, West Hartford, CT 06117, USA; [g] Division of Physical Therapy, School of Health and Rehabilitation Sciences, The Ohio State University, Columbus, OH 43210, USA
* Corresponding author. Cincinnati Children's Hospital, 3333 Burnet Avenue, MLC 10001, Cincinnati, OH 45229.
E-mail address: mark.paterno@cchmc.org

Clin Sports Med 33 (2014) 353–374
http://dx.doi.org/10.1016/j.csm.2014.01.001
0278-5919/14/$ – see front matter © 2014 Elsevier Inc. All rights reserved.

sportsmed.theclinics.com

instability and disruption of adjacent articular cartilage that may result in premature osteoarthritis. OCD lesions are most commonly reported in the knee joint, but they are also known to occur in other joints including the ankle and elbow. Physical therapy has a key role in the management of OCD lesions across the spectrum of nonoperative, preoperative, or postoperative phases of care. This article provides an overview of the role of physical therapy throughout the spectrum of care for patients with OCD lesions.

Role of Physical Therapy in Nonoperative Management of OCD

OCD is an increasingly common cause of joint pain and dysfunction among children, adolescents, and young adults.[4] The long-term sequelae of juvenile OCD may be further joint damage and premature development of osteoarthritis.[2,4–6] In skeletally immature patients, management of OCD lesions of the knee, elbow, and ankle may include a course of nonoperative care if the surrounding articular cartilage is intact and there are no signs of fragmentation or instability of the progeny bone.[4,7,8] Such lesions often present with an insidious onset of activity-related pain, swelling, and tenderness to palpation.[7–12] These lesions may also present with loss of range of motion (ROM), which is likely attributed to pain or swelling as opposed to a loose body resulting in a mechanical block. It is not common for these patients to experience locking of the joint.[8] Various studies suggest a healing rate between 26% and 66%,[1,13,14] with much of the variability attributed to size, location, and severity of the lesion.[14] If a nonoperative course is appropriate, a phased progression toward the previous level of function is recommended to allow for protection of healing tissues while addressing potential impairments present in these patients. These potential impairments include pain, effusion, weakness and altered joint mechanics and movement patterns with activity. Coinciding with these impairments, altered functional capacity and activity tolerance may result. Modifications to this phased rehabilitation progression are indicated depending on the lesion characteristics (ie, size and location), integrity of the surrounding articular cartilage surfaces, and severity of associated impairments.[15,16]

Because of the high risk of progression of OCD, patient and family education regarding activity restrictions are important immediate interventions in the nonoperative management. Mihara and colleagues[8] in 2009 evaluated the nonoperative management of 39 youth baseball players. On follow-up at an average of 14.4 months it was determined that 3 of the 4 patients who showed radiographic evidence of lesion progression had gone against medical advice and continued to throw. A second study by Takahara and colleagues[17] in 2007 found that patients treated nonoperatively for elbow OCD who continued to stress the affected elbow had significantly worse radiographic findings. Therefore, a period of rest and activity restriction is indicated to promote optimal outcomes with nonoperative management; however, there is a lack of consensus as to the appropriate duration. Restrictions are reported in the literature anywhere from 6 to 16 weeks.[6,8,11,14,18] Furthermore, a nonoperative management trial in patients with stable lesions, open growth plates, and no significant loss of ROM may been recommended in the literature for up to 6 months.[7,8,17–19]

Progression of the young individual through phases of treatment, from initial presentation to return to activity, are based on the characteristics of the lesion (ie, size, location, status of surrounding tissue), the understanding of joint biomechanics, and the tissue properties that contribute to the healing of the lesion and surrounding tissues. Criteria for progression as well as a general timeline have been provided but should only be used as a guideline (**Tables 1** and **2**). In general, studies show that juvenile OCD lesions with intact articular cartilage have the greatest healing potential without surgical intervention.[20–22] A comprehensive rehabilitation program and plan of care is developed on an individual basis to maximize outcomes. Typical impairments in this population include a need for restricted weight bearing and/or immobilization to allow for healing, reduced lower extremity strength, altered neuromuscular control, and altered lower extremity movement patterns.[23] Early entry into physical therapy can safely address associated impairments and protect the healing structures, and then appropriately advance the individual toward return to previous functional activities. If at any time a patient undergoing nonoperative treatment experiences increased pain, a loss of ROM, or symptoms such as locking or catching, a physician referral is warranted to evaluate the potential for a progression of intra-articular disorder. Other signs and symptoms such as recalcitrant swelling or new-onset swelling that persists for greater than 72 hours should prompt communication with a physician, because these are additional signs of potential lesion progression.

Table 1
Criteria for phase progression

Phase	Knee	Elbow	Ankle
Progression from acute phase to intermediate phase	No pain No effusion ROM 0°–120° Pain-free weight bearing LE MMT 4 out of 5	No pain No swelling Full ROM	No pain No effusion Full ROM Pain-free weight bearing
Progression to advanced phase	No pain No effusion Full ROM Pain-free FWB with normal gait pattern MMT 4+ out of 5 for hip, knee, and core musculature Normal mechanics during SLS activities	80% of shoulder and elbow strength on noninvolved side	5 out of 5 MMT ankle DF, IV, EV 4 out of 5 MMT ankle PF Pain-free FWB with normal gait pattern 100% SLS of noninvolved limb on stable surface
Progression to return to sport/return to activity reintegration	No pain No effusion Full ROM Pain-free FWB with normal gait pattern MMT 5 out of 5 for hip, knee, and core musculature Isokinetic quadriceps index >85% of contralateral limb Normal mechanics during SLS and impact activities Limb symmetry index >90% on single-leg hop testing	90% of shoulder and elbow strength on noninvolved side Weight-bearing athletes: ability to bear weight through involved upper extremity only without pain Throwing athletes: pain-free unilateral plyometrics	5 out of 5 MMT ankle DF, IV, EV, PF 100% SLS of noninvolved limb on unstable surface

Abbreviations: DF, dorsiflexion; EV, eversion; FWB, full weight bearing; IV, inversion; LE, lower extremity; MMT, manual muscle testing; PF, plant flexion; SLS, single-limb stance.

Table 2
Potential timelines for postoperative phases

Phase	Knee	Elbow	Ankle
Phase I (acute phase)	Cell based • Day 1–week 6 Structural • Day 1–week 4	Microfracture • Day 1–week 4 Structural • Day 1–week 6	Microfracture • Day 1–week 6 Structural • Day 1–week 8
Phase II (intermediate phase)	Cell based • Weeks 6–12 Structural • Weeks 4–8	Microfracture • Weeks 4–8 Structural • Weeks 6–12	Microfracture • Weeks 6–8 Structural • Weeks 8–10
Phase III (advanced phase)	Cell based • Weeks 12–26 Structural • Weeks 8–12	Microfracture • Weeks 8–12 Structural • Weeks 12–16	Microfracture • Weeks 8–12 Structural • Weeks 10–16
Phase IV (return to sport transition)	Cell based • Weeks 26–40+ Structural • Weeks 12–16+	Microfracture • Week 12 onward Structural • Weeks 16 onward	Microfracture • Week 12 onward Structural • Weeks 16 onward
Phase V (sport reintegration)	Cell based • Months 9–18 Structural • Months 4–9	Microfracture • Months 4–6 Structural • Months 6–12	Microfracture • Months 4–6 Structural • Months 6–12

The use of timelines to progress patients through their postoperative rehabilitation are used solely as a guideline to ensure sufficient time for healing. The ultimate progression through each phase is determined solely by attainment of phase specific goals.

Nonoperative Rehabilitation of OCD of the Knee: Initial Phase

Nonoperative management of OCD lesions of the knee is based in the principles of general knee rehabilitation.[15,16] Throughout the rehabilitation progression, protection of the healing tissue is a priority. At first, this may include a period of restricted weight bearing and immobilization.[4] Allowing 4 to 6 weeks of non–weight bearing decreases the compressive forces on the knee and allows a period of rest from weight-bearing stress in patients with tibiofemoral joint lesions.[24] Immobilization is also suggested as a means to protect a healing lesion,[4] and has been recommended through either cylinder cast immobilization[6] or through the use of bracing.[4] Other clinicians recommend the use of an unloader brace in an attempt to selectively decrease compressive forces through the medial or lateral knee joint compartment, depending on the location of the lesion.[4,14] Isolated lesions in the patellofemoral joint are typically permitted to progress weight bearing and mobilization earlier in rehabilitation because of the absence of compressive forces on the site of the lesion with these activities.

Early rehabilitation interventions are often targeted at maintenance of normal mobility at the knee joint and various attempts to improve muscle activation, retain residual muscle strength, and enhance lower extremity neuromuscular control. ROM interventions in the initial phase of rehabilitation focus on return to normal lower extremity mobility, at the conclusion of any potential period of immobilization. Impaired strength and muscle performance are typically addressed with muscle activation interventions such as neuromuscular electrical stimulation,[25] volitional muscular activation tasks, and an incorporation of both open and closed kinetic chain lower extremity strength interventions. Furthermore, an addition of balance and proprioception interventions can enhance lower extremity stability at this phase of rehabilitation.

Nonoperative Rehabilitation of OCD of the Knee: Intermediate Phase

The intermediate phase of nonoperative management of OCD lesions of the knee should focus on progression of targeted interventions. Any period of immobilization has typically resolved and the patient is able to resume normal ambulation. Interventions to address potential gait deviations such as quadriceps reduction gait[26] or frontal plane malalignments should be addressed as the patient advances toward full weight bearing. Gait retraining, which allows for a progression of lower extremity joint loading, is indicated at this time as weight-bearing restrictions are lifted. An attempt to retrain normal arthrokinematics during gait after this injury is critical to minimize abnormal loading of the knee joint.

A primary focus of the intermediate phase it to target residual strength and muscle activation impairments and prepare for an initiation of sports-specific maneuvers. A mix of both open kinetic chain interventions that can target areas of isolated muscle weakness, in addition to closed kinetic exercises that encourage a dynamic incorporation of the lower extremity working to execute a movement pattern is ideal.[6,27] Failure to address isolated weakness can result in abnormal movements patterns with baseline activities[28] as well as with more high-level tasks. If a patient has difficulty activating their quadriceps musculature early after the immobilization period, neuromuscular stimulation or biofeedback can be used to enhance muscle recruitment. A focus on core muscle strength can be advanced during this phase to ensure that athletes will have sufficient core strength[15] to control the movement of their centers of mass during later progressions to dynamic movement patterns. In addition, interventions focused on the development of balance and proprioception are critical because these impairments typically persist after periods of immobilization after injury.[15,16] Once a patient has achieved baseline goals, including resolution of pain, absence of knee effusion, progression of lower extremity strength to a minimum of 4+ out of 5 on a manual muscle test and demonstration of proper mechanics with open and closed kinetic chain exercises, they are progressed to the advanced phase of rehabilitation.[23]

Nonoperative Rehabilitation of OCD of the Knee: Advanced Phase

The goal of the advanced phase of rehabilitation is to build on the foundation of strength and normalization of movement patterns developed in the initial and intermediate phases of rehabilitation with the ultimate goal to advance back to the patient's desired level of activity. Continued progression of advanced strengthening is necessary at this time to address any underlying strength impairments. Advanced strengthening may include a variety of progressions. Most simply, a progression of the weight or volume of activity performed can be incorporated. More dynamically, this may include an incorporation of more functional movement patterns, as well as an advancement of the amount of stability provided by providing an unstable surface to encourage athletes to rely more on their core musculature and proprioceptive skills to stabilize their centers of mass during dynamic movement patterns.

A greater focus of the advanced phase of rehabilitation is to maximize the neuromuscular control of the athlete. Altered movement patterns during dynamic athletic activity have previously been identified as predictors of various lower extremity injuries not only in healthy athletes[29] but also in athletes attempting to return from injury.[30] As a result, interventions that focus on normalizing movement patterns, encouraging symmetry between lower extremities, and replicating anticipated movements required for future desired activities by the patients are critical. A typical progression during the advanced stage of rehabilitation may include an increased focus on single-limb activities or an initiation of light-impact activities. For each of these progressions, the main focus should initially be on technique. A patient who previously experienced knee pain with isolated movements or at specific angles of knee flexion, which is typical with an isolated OCD lesion, may continue to show abnormal movement patterns to avoid a painful ROM (**Fig. 1**). Regular feedback is necessary to retrain normal movement patterns and reduce the risk of potential future injury. Progression to impact loading is indicated in those individuals who will return to impact sports, but a graduated reintegration is necessary to protect the healing tissues. Light plyometric activity with restricted volume to start can ultimately be progressed to higher volume activity over time as tolerated by the patient as long as there is no risk to healing tissue. Once patients have reached the goals of the final stage of rehabilitation, which include normal mobility, normal lower extremity strength (limb symmetry index greater than 85%), normal neuromuscular control indicated by no abnormal movement with dynamic tasks, and absence of pain and effusion, they are ready to transition to a return to sport/return to activity program that best meets their individual goals.[23]

Nonoperative Rehabilitation of OCD of the Elbow: Acute Phase

The goals of the first phase of nonoperative elbow rehabilitation are to decrease pain and swelling and restore full ROM while minimizing complications of inactivity. It may be appropriate initially to restrict ROM during this phase to protect the involved joint. A hinged brace may be used at the elbow to limit painful ROM. Some investigators have recommended an offloader brace during nonoperative management to allow a quicker return to pain-free activity.[11]

In order to decrease pain and swelling, joint mobilizations, passive ROM, and modalities such as cryotherapy and electrical stimulation may be used during this phase. Joint mobilizations may also be indicated to increase ROM along with active and passive ROM exercises as tolerated. To minimize the effects of inactivity, proprioception and isometric exercises at the involved joint may be initiated. In addition, strengthening of the core and proximal musculature as well as cardiovascular conditioning using a stationary bike or elliptical trainer is appropriate. All exercises during this phase should be performed in a non–weight-bearing position for the involved joint to avoid excessive compression and shear forces. Progression to the intermediate phase is indicated when the patient presents without pain or swelling and with full ROM.

Nonoperative Rehabilitation of OCD of the Elbow: Intermediate Phase

The goals of the intermediate phase are to initiate isotonic strengthening at the involved joint and progress general strengthening of joints proximal and distal to the elbow. All strengthening exercises in this phase should again be performed in a non–weight-bearing position. Patients with OCD of the elbow may begin to use the upper body ergometer during this phase. To minimize the effects of exercise-induced soreness, appropriate modalities may be used during this and the subsequent phases. Progression to the next phase is indicated when the patient shows shoulder and elbow strength of at least 80% of the contralateral side.

Nonoperative Rehabilitation of OCD of the Elbow: Advanced Phase

For patients with OCD of the elbow, the advanced phase is a progressive strengthening phase with initiation of weight-bearing or plyometric exercises to prepare the patient to return to sport. A systematic progression of both weight-bearing and plyometric activities should be implemented. Weight-bearing exercises should be initiated

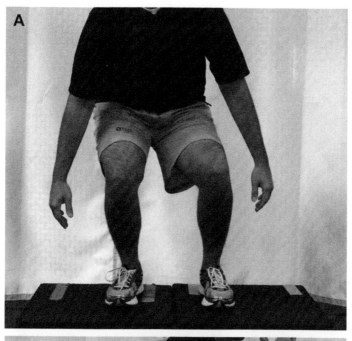

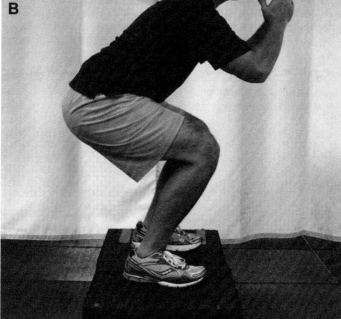

Fig. 1. (*A*) A squat with unloading of the involved limb. (*B*) A squat with equal distribution of force between limbs.

in a bilateral position with modified weight (**Fig. 2**) and can be progressed to full weight bearing on the involved extremity only. Plyometrics can also be progressed from bilateral to unilateral exercises.

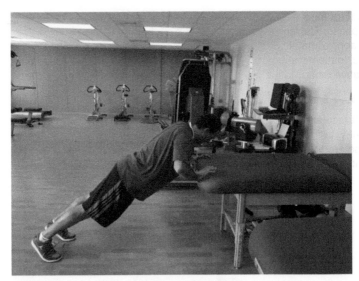

Fig. 2. Modified weight bearing: push up on table.

For elbow OCD, the patient may progress to the return-to-sport phase of rehabilitation when 90% of the strength at the uninvolved shoulder and elbow is achieved. It is also recommended that patients who will return to weight-bearing activities, such as gymnastics or wrestling, show the ability to bear weight through the involved upper extremity in an isolated fashion without pain. Patients who will return to throwing activities should show pain-free unilateral plyometric activities such as those seen in **Fig. 3**.

Nonoperative Rehabilitation of OCD of the Elbow: Return-to Sport Phase

During the final phase of rehabilitation the athletes should participate in sport-specific activities. In addition to ongoing strengthening and progressive weight-bearing

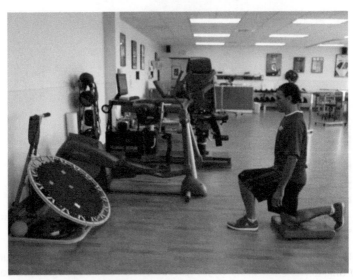

Fig. 3. Unilateral plyometrics: half-kneel ball toss.

activities (**Fig. 4**), overhead athletes should initiate an interval-throwing program during this phase. Current evidence suggests that interval-throwing programs should begin at approximately 3 to 4 months during a nonoperative rehabilitation program.[8] Therefore, patients should enter the final phase after approximately 3 months of nonoperative rehabilitation for OCD of the elbow.

Nonoperative Management of OCD of the Ankle: Acute Phase

The fundamental principles guiding nonoperative management of ankle OCD are consistent with those seen in patients with knee and elbow lesions. The goals of the first phase are to decrease pain and swelling and restore full ROM while minimizing complications of inactivity. It may be appropriate initially to restrict ROM during this

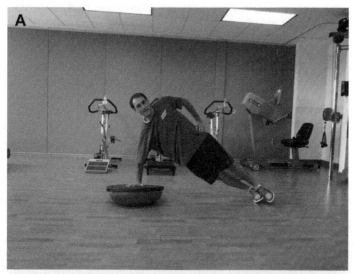

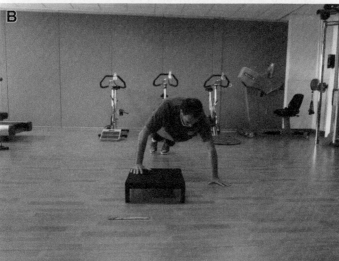

Fig. 4. (*A*) Unilateral weight bearing with perturbations: side plank on BOSU. (*B*) Weight bearing with impact: walk over 15-cm step.

phase to protect the involved joint. For nonoperative management of OCD at the ankle, limited weight bearing may be required in addition to limited ROM. Some investigators have recommended use of a short leg cast or walking boot for a period of 3 to 8 weeks.[12] However, a walking boot is preferred rather than a short leg cast to allow controlled motion at the involved ankle joint, which is critical to promote movement of synovial fluid and facilitate joint nutrition. Similar to other joints, a joint protection program is initiated while attempting to progress proximal and core musculature strength. Cardiovascular endurance activity can be initiated with the use of an upper body ergometer as tolerated.

Progression to the next phase is indicated when the patient presents with full ROM and no reports of pain or swelling. In addition, patients should show the ability to bear weight through the involved ankle without pain. Patients may spend approximately 6 weeks in the acute phase to allow adequate physiologic healing before advancement of weight-bearing activity.

Nonoperative Rehabilitation of OCD of the Ankle: Intermediate Phase

The goals of the intermediate phase are to initiate isotonic strengthening at the involved joint and progress general strengthening of joints proximal and distal to the lesion and facilitate a normal gait pattern. Similar to OCD of the knee, static stretching of the involved lower extremity may be performed in weight bearing along with static single-limb stance proprioceptive training to help normalize gait patterns. Use of the stationary bike and elliptical trainer may begin during this phase. Progression to the next phase is indicated when the patient presents with 5/5 for manual muscle testing of all ankle muscles except for 4/5 for plantar flexion, ambulates all distances without antalgic gait, and performs static single-limb stance on a stable surface 100% of contralateral limb time.

Nonoperative Rehabilitation of OCD of the Ankle: Advanced Phase

Patients with OCD of the ankle should progress toward more advanced closed chain strengthening of the lower extremities during this phase (**Fig. 5**). Balance should be progressed to dynamic activities incorporating perturbation training to prepare the athlete for sport-specific demands (**Fig. 6**). Progression to the final phase of rehabilitation is indicated when normal strength of all involved ankle musculature is present and the patient is able to show 100% of single-limb stance balance and stability on an unstable surface compared with the uninvolved side.

Nonoperative Rehabilitation of OCD of the Ankle: Return-to-sport Phase

In an attempt to appropriately progress back to weight-bearing athletic activity, patients should progress weight-bearing activities to incorporate elements of added difficulty such as perturbations or impact to best reflect the specific demands of the sport. Patients may initiate treadmill running as well as advanced plyometrics and agility drills using a bilateral to unilateral progression. Activity restrictions have been cited in the literature for 3 to 4 months for nonoperative management of OCD at the ankle,[9,12] therefore return to sports activities typically occurs within this time frame.

Skeletal maturity, early diagnosis of a low-grade lesion, ROM, and type and level of sport have all been cited as factors affecting the ability to successfully treat elbow OCDs nonoperatively.[8,11,17] However, there is a lack of consensus as to the optimal duration of conservative management of these OCDs. Literature has recommended anywhere from 3 to 8 months of nonoperative rehabilitation before return to sport.[8,10,12,19] It is therefore recommended that rehabilitation professionals monitor patient status for significant changes in presentation while implementing a protocol with

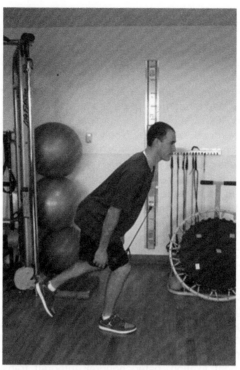

Fig. 5. Advanced closed kinetic chain strengthening: bird dip.

criteria for progression that are tailored toward the sport-specific needs of each patient. Successful completion of an interval-throwing program or adequate demonstration of weight-bearing or plyometric tasks mimicking sport-specific demands should indicate safe return to previous level of function after nonoperative rehabilitation.

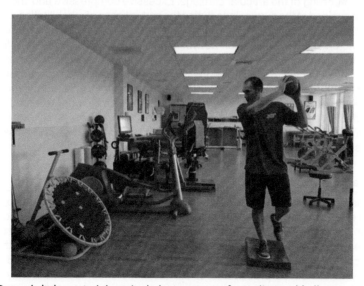

Fig. 6. Dynamic balance training: single-leg stance on foam diagonal ball toss.

Role of Physical Therapy in Operative Management of OCD

Operative management of osteochondritis dissecans lesions may be necessary in various cases.

The presence of unstable lesions, articular cartilage involvement, skeletal maturity, or failure of nonoperative management may result in the need for surgical management. Signs and symptoms of unstable lesions include insidious onset of activity-related pain, stiffness, and tenderness to palpation at the joint line along with locking, catching, and limited ROM.[7,8,10,11,17,31–33] Surgical management of OCD lesions can be dichotomized into procedures involving only subchondral bone and those involving both subchondral bone and articular cartilage. Physical therapy interventions are unique for each of these groups of procedures because of the native tissues affected.

Surgical interventions focused only on subchondral bone are indicated when the articular cartilage is intact and the subchondral bone has failed to heal with a non-operative course of treatment. In this case, the global aim of the surgical intervention is to stimulate the subchondral bone growth. This stimulation can be obtained through a drilling procedure[34,35] or a drilling procedure augmented with bone graft.[36] One of the most concerning indications for surgery is the presence of an OCD with involvement of articular cartilage. Because of the reduced healing potential of articular cartilage, these injuries have the potential to progress to early osteoarthritis. Surgical management of articular cartilage injury is evolving with the optimal surgical intervention often depending on factors such as the size of the lesion, extent of involvement of the articular cartilage, and the location of the lesion. Procedures involving the subchondral bone and articular cartilage can be further subdivided into structural procedures and cell-based procedures. Structural interventions include procedures such as osteochondral fragment fixation, osteochondral autograft transplants, and osteochondral allograft transplants. Cell-based interventions include procedures that attempt to stimulate regrowth of cartilage tissue. These procedures may include microfracture, marrow stimulation, and autologous chondrocyte implantation (ACI) procedures.[37]

Postoperative rehabilitation should provide an environment that allows safe adaptation and remodeling of the articular cartilage. Excessive compressive and shear forces need to be avoided at the surgical site during the early phases of rehabilitation. Similar to nonoperative rehabilitation protocols, the postoperative protocols are divided into phases with criteria for progression between each phase. However, there is little evidence in the literature validating optimal rehabilitation interventions for patients with operative management of OCD lesions. Therefore, rehabilitation progressions are based on the basic science of healing tissue and the underlying goal to implement interventions known to address comparable impairments in similar populations. Timelines are provided in **Table 2** but should be used only as guidelines. A progression of interventions from initial postsurgical management through return to activity is discussed with highlights on necessary modification for each subclassification of surgical intervention.

Postoperative Rehabilitation of Knee OCD: Acute Phase

The primary goals of the acute postoperative phase are to manage postoperative pain and effusion while introducing exercises to progress ROM, strength, and neuro-muscular control. Patients begin with a non–weight-bearing ambulation status to allow adequate healing after surgery. Patients with structural procedures in the tibio-femoral compartment commonly have restricted weight bearing for 4 to 6 weeks. Patients with cell-based procedures of the tibiofemoral compartment may have a prolonged period of restricted weight bearing for 6 to 8 weeks. All patellofemoral procedures typically undergo a 2-week to 4-week period of restricted weight bearing. In addition, patellofemoral procedures may also use postoperative ROM bracing to control knee flexion and protect the patellofemoral joint, which may not be necessary with tibiofemoral lesions.

The initial rehabilitation focus with any procedure involving articular cartilage needs to include early mobility.[15] Patients with operative management of tibiofemoral lesions and structural interventions of patellofemoral lesions, such as osteochondral fragment fixation, present with no ROM restrictions after surgery. Patients with cell-based management of patellofemoral lesions may present with an initial protected ROM for the first 2 to 4 weeks after surgery, depending on the size of the lesion.[38] With respect to interventions to enhance mobility and promote articular cartilage health, continuous active assisted and passive motion is advocated immediately after surgery. This immediate motion helps the patients to deter knee stiffness but also promotes synovial fluid circulation and fosters intra-articular nutrition throughout the knee joint. Some controversy exists over the use of mechanical continuous passive motion (CPM) versus simply using patient-guided passive motion,[39] but all agree that immediate and frequent motion is necessary to facilitate normal mobility and joint health in this population.

The initiation of interventions to deter disuse atrophy and facilitate a progression of muscle activation and strength begins within the acute phase of rehabilitation. Knee joint–specific interventions must focus on quadriceps muscle activation. If muscle activation is limited because of postoperative effusion and pain, modalities are indicated to address these impairments. The use of cryotherapy to target joint effusion and pain, as well as neuromuscular stimulation to facilitate a more rapid return of muscle activation early after surgical intervention,[25] may be indicated. More regionally, strengthening interventions that focus on both the hip and ankle joints as well as interventions that target core stability can be initiated early after surgery.[15,16,27] The primary guideline for early progression of these exercises is within the patient's weight-bearing status, because this often limits the ability to progress to closed kinetic chain exercises. Once patients have achieved baseline goals, inclusive of minimal pain and effusion, appropriate ROM and good quadriceps activation, they are ready to progress to the intermediate phase of rehabilitation.

Postoperative Rehabilitation of Knee OCD: Intermediate Phase

The focus in the intermediate phase of rehabilitation is on the initiation of more advanced neuromuscular control and balance/proprioception interventions, while continuing to advance lower extremity and core strengthening exercises. The patient may continue to present with weight-bearing restrictions that can limit progression of weight-bearing activities[27]; however, once the patient is fully weight bearing, without restriction, there is an opportunity to advance dynamic functional training and progressive joint loading activities. Interventions that focus on balance and proprioception retraining are indicated at this time to enhance position sense around the knee joint.[15,16] In addition, a focus on neuromuscular control with continual feedback to both guide the technique and facilitate appropriate symmetry of joint loading is critical at this time. The development of abnormal movement patterns during the initial weight-bearing interventions have the potential to carry over into higher level activities. An early focus on technique and a slow progression of joint loading are key focus areas in the intermediate phase of rehabilitation. When the patient shows progression of strength and muscle activation with a baseline skill of symmetric joint loading, while still presenting with no pain or effusion, it is appropriate to move toward the advanced stage of rehabilitation.

Postoperative Rehabilitation of Knee OCD: Advanced Phase

After a surgical intervention to manage OCD of the knee, the advanced postoperative phase of rehabilitation prepares patients for a return to preinjury and sports activities. During this phase, the goal is to maximize strengthening interventions to resolve any residual strength impairments while appropriately progressing joint loading interventions consistent with the patient goals. If the patient desires a return to an impact loading activity, clinical experts suggest that this is an appropriate time to introduce and progress plyometric activity, despite not being well defined in the literature.[16] In general, limited evidence exists for an optimal time frame to return to impact activity. Criteria for progression to impact have been outlined by Wilk and colleagues[16] and others, but this remains expert opinion. It is recommended that an introduction to impact activity is not initiated until a minimum of 3 months following any structural intervention and between 3 and 6 months for any cell-based intervention. Impact progression should begin with low-impact, single-plane, bipedal tasks and eventually progress to more single-limb, triplanar tasks. Low-impact activity such as hopping and light jogging can be progressed in intensity with more advanced plyometric activity movements. In addition, therapists should provide regular verbal and tactile feedback, focused on developing appropriate technique.[40] Feedback should facilitate normal movement patterns and deter any of the potential limb asymmetries that are often seen with unilateral injury (**Figs. 7** and **8**).[28] Once the patient has achieved normal strength parameters (typically reported to be 85%–90% of the contralateral limb[41–43]) and has successfully completed a functional progression through impact loading activity, enrollment in a return-to-sport/return-to-activity program is indicated before ultimate discharge. A typical time frame necessary for a patient to successfully achieve all return-to-sport criteria following an operative intervention for OCD of the knee can range from 3 to 6 months with structural procedures and 4 to 18 months for cell-based procedures, depending on size and location of lesion as well as other perioperative factors.

Postoperative Rehabilitation of OCD of the Elbow

Operative interventions to address OCD of the elbow may include either structural or cell-based interventions. Cell-based procedures include ACI (autologous chondrocyte transplantation) and bone marrow stimulation procedures (such as microfracture). However, ACI is not yet widely practiced as a surgical intervention for OCD of the elbow and therefore is not included in the postoperative elbow protocol. Structural repairs include osteochondral transplantation, both autograft and allograft, and OCD fixation.

Postoperative Rehabilitation of Elbow OCD: Acute Phase

The goals of the acute phase are to eliminate postoperative sequelae, increase ROM, and minimize the secondary effects of inactivity. Manual therapy is indicated during this phase to decrease pain and swelling and promote scar and joint mobility. Therapeutic exercises such as active ROM of the surrounding joints are encouraged along with proximal strengthening as tolerated. Isometric contractions across the involved joint may be initiated for both cellular and structural procedures. Isotonic contractions can be performed after microfracture and debridement procedures after the first 2 weeks to allow for formation of the fibrin clot and granulation tissue.[44] Cardiovascular conditioning may be performed on the appropriate equipment to maintain a non–weight-bearing status of the elbow, because all exercises during this phase should be performed in a non–weight-bearing position. Modalities such as cryotherapy and electrical stimulation are indicated to decrease postoperative pain and swelling.

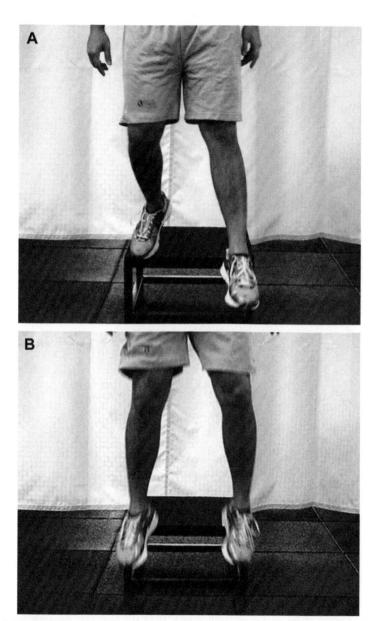

Fig. 7. (A) Patient takeoff during a drop landing task. Note the significant limb asymmetry as the patient leads with the uninvolved limb in an attempt to unweight the involved limb. (B) Patient takeoff during a drop landing task with appropriate limb symmetry noted at takeoff.

Mixed evidence suggests immobilization after structural repair at the elbow for 2 to 3 weeks of the acute phase in a long arm cast. If a cast is used, physical therapy is initiated following cast removal.[31,33,45] An alternative to casting can be a hinged brace during this phase to restrict ROM to a pain-free range and to allow immediate controlled mobility at the joint.

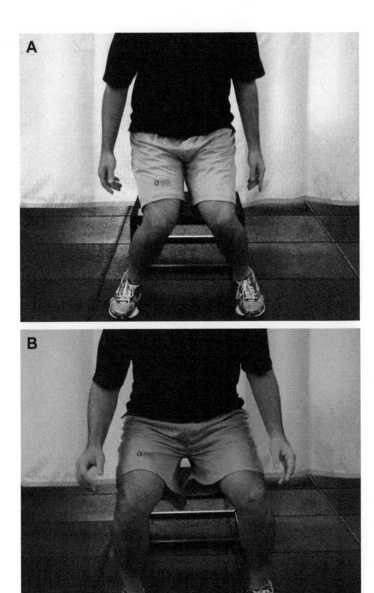

Fig. 8. (*A*) Landing phase of a drop landing task. Note the high-risk, dynamic valgus positioning at landing. This position is known to be a risk factor for anterior cruciate ligament injury but also results in asymmetric distribution of force through the knee joint during landing. (*B*) Landing phase of the drop landing task with good lower extremity alignment.

Postoperative Rehabilitation of Elbow OCD: Intermediate Phase and Advanced Phase

Progression to the intermediate phase occurs after postoperative pain and swelling have subsided and full ROM has been achieved. The emphasis during the intermediate and advanced phases of rehabilitation is on progressive strengthening. It is expected that patients need a minimum of 6 weeks to allow for adaptive strengthening to occur. Patients after structural repair are likely to spend close to 10 to 12 weeks in this process. Initiation of weight-bearing or plyometric exercises in the advanced phase may begin when the patient shows involved shoulder and elbow strength of at least 80% of the uninvolved side.

Progression to the final phase should be restricted until the patient shows 90% of the uninvolved upper extremity shoulder and elbow strength on the involved side. Functional tasks specific to the demands of the sport, such as the ability to bear weight through the involved upper extremity in an isolated fashion without pain or pain-free plyometric activities, should also be assessed.

Postoperative Rehabilitation of Elbow OCD: Return-to-sport Phase

During the final phase of rehabilitation, athletes should initiate participation in sport-specific activities. For patients who will be returning to throwing, an interval-throwing program should be introduced during this phase. The literature supports a general timeline for transitioning patients into this phase. Because of the presence of fibrocartilage and hyaline cartilage as well as restored subchondral bone during weeks 12 to 48,[44] it is recommended that patients delay progression to sport until a minimum of 3 to 4 months after microfracture. Care should be taken to delay this phase in patients who have undergone a structural repair to allow for adequate graft incorporation. A study by Iwasaki and colleagues[31] in 2009 found graft incorporation on MRI in most patients 6 months after autologous osteochondral mosaicplasty at the elbow. Therefore, it is recommended that patients after structural repair return to sport-specific activities at approximately months 5 to 6.[7,31,33]

Postoperative Rehabilitation of Ankle OCD: Acute Phase

Progression of weight bearing is a concern during the acute phase of rehabilitation after operative management of ankle OCDs. Weight-bearing status after microfracture and chondroplasty varies in the literature from full weight bearing immediately to 8 weeks after surgery.[44] It is our recommendation that patients who undergo a microfracture or chondroplasty procedure maintain a non–weight-bearing status for at least 2 weeks to allow for formation of a fibrin clot.[44] Partial weight bearing may be progressed beginning at week 2. Full weight bearing is allowed after 6 to 8 weeks as fibrocartilaginous tissue is formed. For structural repairs, the literature varies from partial weight bearing at weeks 0 to 6[46] to non–weight bearing for the first 4 weeks followed by partial weight bearing for the remaining 4 weeks,[47] which is our recommendation to minimize stress during the initial phases of bone healing. Progression to the next phase is indicated when the patient presents with no pain, minimal swelling, and full ROM. Patients should also show the ability to bear weight through the involved lower extremity without pain.

Postoperative Rehabilitation of Ankle OCD: Intermediate and Advanced Phase

The primary focus during these phases is progression of stability, mobility, and strength. Patients may discontinue the use of any brace once adequate protective strength is achieved. Impairments should be addressed to allow the patient to ambulate all distances without an antalgic gait. Therapeutic exercises should focus on building strength and flexibility of the core and involved extremity. Proprioception training should also be addressed during this phase including weight shifting and static single-limb stance activities on a stable surface **Fig. 9**. Patients with ankle OCD may transition to the advanced phase when the patient presents with 5 out of 5 manual testing of all ankle muscles except for 4 out of 5 plantar flexion, ambulation all distances without antalgic gait, and ability to perform static single-limb stance on a

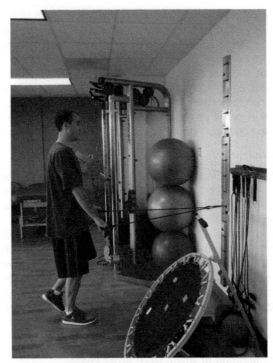

Fig. 9. Single-limb stance on a stable surface with weight shifting.

stable surface 100% of contralateral limb time. During the advanced phase, therapeutic activities should progress in difficulty to incorporate dynamic balance and perturbation training in addition to ongoing strengthening.

Postoperative Rehabilitation of Ankle OCD: Return-to-sport Phase

Patients after ankle OCD surgery may initiate return to sport activities on demonstration of 5 out of 5 ankle strength in all planes and 100% of single-limb stance on an unstable surface compared with the contralateral side. Patients who will be returning to running and cutting sports should initiate a gradual return-to-running program and plyometric and agility drills progressing from bilateral to unilateral activities. Similar to patients with OCD of the knee, this should be a graduated progression to systematically introduce and progress impact and joint loading forces. The initiation of return to impact activities may begin a minimum of 4 to 6 months after surgery.

Postoperative Rehabilitation of Ankle OCD: Ankle ACI

Postoperative management of OCD at the ankle with the use of ACI is more conservative than microfracture at this joint because the biological evidence suggests that ACI procedures require a longer timeline for healing. Most published ACI rehabilitation literature has examined the knee; however, patients with ACI at the ankle joint are likely to have to progress more slowly than patients with ACI at the knee because of the increased joint congruity of the ankle.[48] There are no controlled studies that report on clinical outcomes following ACI of the ankle according to a meta-analysis by Niemeyer and colleagues[48] in 2012. The published literature makes little reference to postoperative protocols, and the recommendations made are inconsistent. Rehabilitation should therefore use the previously discussed postoperative phases. Care should be taken to progress slowly through the postoperative phases during the first 3 months, because the repair site is most vulnerable during that time.[49,50]

The first 6 weeks is referred to in the literature as the proliferative stage.[49,51] During this stage, immediate passive ROM is a consistent recommendation supported in the literature to minimize postoperative sequelae and assist in cellular orientation.[49–55] Weight-bearing status varies during this phase from progressive weight bearing as tolerated[54] to non–weight bearing for 6 to 8 weeks.[52,53] Taking into account the significant congruity at the talocrural joint during weight bearing and the need to protect the graft, progression to weight bearing and other activities that place shear stress on the graft should be limited for at least 6 weeks.

During the transition stage of healing, care should be taken to gradually introduce and progress weight-bearing exercises because weight bearing helps to stimulate cartilage maturation.[51,56] After 3 to 6 months, the repair tissue is well integrated to the underlying bone and adjacent cartilage[49] and therefore progression to the next phase of activities is appropriate.

Graft remodeling and maturation may take more than 2 years after implantation.[49,50] However, initiation of the final phase of activities may begin at approximately months 6 to 9 because of the significant improvement in cartilage remodeling.[49,55] This recommendation is consistent with previously published guidelines at the knee.[50,55] A study specific to ACI at the talus by Baums and colleagues[52] in 2006 allowed patients to initiate running at 6 months and reported good to excellent results in 11 out of 12 patients. Cherubino and colleagues[53] in 2003 allowed patients to return to low-level activity such as swimming and cycling at 3 months, but restricted running, cutting, and jumping for 10 months. It is our recommendation to limit return to sport slightly longer, until months 12 to 18 after ACI at the talus, which is more consistent with published literature at the knee.[49,50]

Sport Reintegration

Postoperative return-to-sport time frames vary depending on the postoperative protocol. The literature has cited return to sport after microfracture from 6 weeks to 6 months after surgery.[7,11,44] Structural repair procedures limit return to sport for anywhere from 6 to 12 months.[7,31] It is the recommendation of these investigators that successful completion of an interval-throwing program or adequate demonstration of weight-bearing tasks mimicking sport-specific demands should indicate safe return to sport following a postoperative rehabilitation program. Successful completion of this phased approach to postoperative rehabilitation typically allows return to sport after microfracture approximately 4 to 6 months after surgery, whereas return to sport is typically 6 to 12 months after structural repair.

Summary

Physical therapy management of osteochondritis dissecans can incorporate a full spectrum of conservative, nonoperative, and postoperative care. Rehabilitation interventions can vary based on factors such as the lesion characteristics, lesion location, articular cartilage involvement, skeletal maturity of the patient, presenting impairments at the time of evaluation, and concomitant injury. It is the responsibility of the rehabilitation professional to address all corresponding factors and mindfully advance the patient with a systematic and evidence-based progression to protect healing tissue and optimize outcome.

REFERENCES

1. Cahill BR. Osteochondritis dissecans of the knee: treatment of juvenile and adult forms. J Am Acad Orthop Surg 1995;3(4):237–47.

2. Detterline AJ, Goldstein JL, Rue JP, et al. Evaluation and treatment of osteo-chondritis dissecans lesions of the knee. J Knee Surg 2008;21(2):106–15.
3. Glancy GL. Juvenile osteochondritis dissecans. Am J Knee Surg 1999;12(2): 120–4.
4. Kocher MS, Tucker R, Ganley TJ, et al. Management of osteochondritis disse-cans of the knee: current concepts review. Am J Sports Med 2006;34(7): 1181–91.
5. Twyman RS, Desai K, Aichroth PM. Osteochondritis dissecans of the knee. A long-term study. J Bone Joint Surg Br 1991;73(3):461–4.
6. Wall E, Von Stein D. Juvenile osteochondritis dissecans. Orthop Clin North Am 2003;34(3):341–53.
7. Greiwe RM, Saifi C, Ahmad CS. Pediatric sports elbow injuries. Clin Sports Med 2010;29(4):677–703.
8. Mihara K, Tsutsui H, Nishinaka N, et al. Nonoperative treatment for osteochon-dritis dissecans of the capitellum. Am J Sports Med 2009;37(2):298–304.
9. deGraaw C. Osteochondral lesion of the talus in a recreational athlete: a case report. J Can Chiropr Assoc 1999;43(1):15.
10. Jones RB, Miller RH. Bony overuse injuries about the elbow. Oper Tech Orthop 2001;11(1):55–62.
11. Savoie FH. Osteochondritis dissecans of the elbow. Oper Tech Sports Med 2008;16(4):187–93.
12. Thacker MM, Dabney KW, Mackenzie WG. Osteochondritis dissecans of the talar head: natural history and review of literature. J Pediatr Orthop B 2012; 21(4):373–6.
13. Parikh SN, Allen M, Wall EJ, et al. The reliability to determine "healing" in osteo-chondritis dissecans from radiographic assessment. J Pediatr Orthop 2012; 32(6):e35–9.
14. Wall EJ, Vourazeris J, Myer GD, et al. The healing potential of stable juvenile osteochondritis dissecans knee lesions. J Bone Joint Surg Am 2008;90(12): 2655–64.
15. Reinold MM, Wilk KE, Macrina LC, et al. Current concepts in the rehabilitation following articular cartilage repair procedures in the knee. J Orthop Sports Phys Ther 2006;36(10):774–94.
16. Wilk KE, Briem K, Reinold MM, et al. Rehabilitation of articular lesions in the athlete's knee. J Orthop Sports Phys Ther 2006;36(10):815–27.
17. Takahara M, Mura N, Sasaki J, et al. Classification, treatment, and outcome of osteochondritis dissecans of the humeral capitellum. J Bone Joint Surg Am 2007;89(6):1205–14.
18. Krabak BJ, Alexander E, Henning T. Shoulder and elbow injuries in the adoles-cent athlete. Phys Med Rehabil Clin N Am 2008;19(2):271–85, viii.
19. Bradley JP, Petrie RS. Osteochondritis dissecans of the humeral capitellum. Diagnosis and treatment. Clin Sports Med 2001;20(3):565–90.
20. De Smet AA, Ilahi OA, Graf BK. Untreated osteochondritis dissecans of the femoral condyles: prediction of patient outcome using radiographic and MR findings. Skeletal Radiol 1997;26(8):463–7.
21. Hughes JA, Cook JV, Churchill MA, et al. Juvenile osteochondritis dissecans: a 5-year review of the natural history using clinical and MRI evaluation. Pediatr Radiol 2003;33(6):410–7.
22. Jurgensen I, Bachmam G, Schleicher I, et al. Osteochondritis dissecans – an easy classification in MRI. Z Orthop Ihre Grenzgeb 2002;140(1):58–64 [in German].

23. Schmitt L, Byrnes R, Cherny C, et al. Cincinnati Children's Hospital Medical Center: evidence-based clinical care guideline for management of osteochondritis dissecans of the knee. 2009. Guideline 037. p. 1–16. Available at: http://www.cincinnatichildrens.org/svc/alpha/h/health-policy/ev-based/otpt.htm. Accessed December 17, 2009.
24. Buckwalter JA. Articular cartilage: injuries and potential for healing. J Orthop Sports Phys Ther 1998;28(4):192–202.
25. Snyder-Mackler L, Delitto A, Bailey SL, et al. Strength of the quadriceps femoris muscle and functional recovery after reconstruction of the anterior cruciate ligament. A prospective, randomized clinical trial of electrical stimulation. J Bone Joint Surg Am 1995;77(8):1166–73.
26. Berchuck M, Andriacchi TP, Bach BR, et al. Gait adaptations by patients who have a deficient anterior cruciate ligament. J Bone Joint Surg Am 1990;72(6):871–7.
27. Ganley TJ, Gaugler RL, Kocher MS, et al. Osteochondritis dissecans of the knee. Oper Tech Sports Med 2006;14(3):147–58.
28. Ernst GP, Saliba E, Diduch DR, et al. Lower extremity compensations following anterior cruciate ligament reconstruction. Phys Ther 2000;80(3):251–60.
29. Hewett TE, Myer GD, Ford KR, et al. Biomechanical measures of neuromuscular control and valgus loading of the knee predict anterior cruciate ligament injury risk in female athletes: a prospective study. Am J Sports Med 2005;33(4):492–501.
30. Paterno MV, Schmitt LC, Ford KR, et al. Biomechanical measures during landing and postural stability predict second anterior cruciate ligament injury after anterior cruciate ligament reconstruction and return to sport. Am J Sports Med 2010;38(10):1968–78.
31. Iwasaki N, Kato H, Kamishima T, et al. Sequential alterations in magnetic resonance imaging findings after autologous osteochondral mosaicplasty for young athletes with osteochondritis dissecans of the humeral capitellum. Am J Sports Med 2009;37(12):2349–54.
32. Schoch B, Wolf BR. Osteochondritis dissecans of the capitellum: minimum 1-year follow-up after arthroscopic debridement. Arthroscopy 2010;26(11):1469–73.
33. Takeda H, Watarai K, Matsushita T, et al. A surgical treatment for unstable osteochondritis dissecans lesions of the humeral capitellum in adolescent baseball players. Am J Sports Med 2002;30(5):713–7.
34. Anderson AF, Richards DB, Pagnani MJ, et al. Antegrade drilling for osteochondritis dissecans of the knee. Arthroscopy 1997;13(3):319–24.
35. Edmonds EW, Albright J, Bastrom T, et al. Outcomes of extra-articular, intra-epiphyseal drilling for osteochondritis dissecans of the knee. J Pediatr Orthop 2010;30(8):870–8.
36. Lykissas MG, Wall EJ, Nathan S. Retro-articular drilling and bone grafting of juvenile knee osteochondritis dissecans: a technical description. Knee Surg Sports Traumatol Arthrosc 2013;22(2):274–8.
37. Magnussen RA, Dunn WR, Carey JL, et al. Treatment of focal articular cartilage defects in the knee: a systematic review. Clin Orthop Relat Res 2008;466(4):952–62.
38. Gobbi A, Kon E, Berruto M, et al. Patellofemoral full-thickness chondral defects treated with second-generation autologous chondrocyte implantation: results at 5 years' follow-up. Am J Sports Med 2009;37(6):1083–92.
39. Knapik DM, Harris JD, Pangrazzi G, et al. The basic science of continuous passive motion in promoting knee health: a systematic review of studies in a rabbit model. Arthroscopy 2013;29(10):1722–31.

40. Gokeler A, Benjaminse A, Hewett TE, et al. Feedback techniques to target functional deficits following anterior cruciate ligament reconstruction: implications for motor control and reduction of second injury risk. Sports Med 2013;43(11): 1065–74.

41. Keays SL, Bullock-Saxton JE, Newcombe P, et al. The relationship between knee strength and functional stability before and after anterior cruciate ligament reconstruction. J Orthop Res 2003;21(2):231–7.

42. Kvist J. Rehabilitation following anterior cruciate ligament injury: current recommendations for sports participation. Sports Med 2004;34(4):269–80.

43. Schmitt LC, Paterno MV, Hewett TE. The impact of quadriceps femoris strength asymmetry on functional performance at return to sport following anterior cruciate ligament reconstruction. J Orthop Sports Phys Ther 2012;42(9):750–9.

44. van Eekeren IC, Reilingh ML, van Dijk CN. Rehabilitation and return-to-sports activity after debridement and bone marrow stimulation of osteochondral talar defects. Sports Med 2012;42(10):857–70.

45. Yamamoto Y, Ishibashi Y, Tsuda E, et al. Osteochondral autograft transplantation for osteochondritis dissecans of the elbow in juvenile baseball players: minimum 2-year follow-up. Am J Sports Med 2006;34(5):714–20.

46. Woelfle JV, Reichel H, Nelitz M. Indications and limitations of osteochondral autologous transplantation in osteochondritis dissecans of the talus. Knee Surg Sports Traumatol Arthrosc 2013;21(8):1925–30.

47. Nakagawa S, Hara K, Minami G, et al. Arthroscopic fixation technique for osteochondral lesions of the talus. Foot Ankle Int 2010;31(11):1025–7.

48. Niemeyer P, Salzmann G, Schmal H, et al. Autologous chondrocyte implantation for the treatment of chondral and osteochondral defects of the talus: a meta-analysis of available evidence. Knee Surg Sports Traumatol Arthrosc 2012; 20(9):1696–703.

49. Hambly K, Bobic V, Wondrasch B, et al. Autologous chondrocyte implantation postoperative care and rehabilitation: science and practice. Am J Sports Med 2006;34(6):1020–38.

50. Riegger-Krugh CL, McCarty EC, Robinson MS, et al. Autologous chondrocyte implantation: current surgery and rehabilitation. Med Sci Sports Exerc 2008; 40(2):206–14.

51. Lewis PB, McCarthy LP, Kang RW, et al. Basic science and treatment options for articular cartilage injuries. J Orthop Sports Phys Ther 2006;36(10):717–27.

52. Baums MH, Heidrich G, Schultz W, et al. Autologous chondrocyte transplantation for treating cartilage defects of the talus. J Bone Joint Surg Am 2006; 88(2):303–8.

53. Cherubino P, Grassi FA, Bulgheroni P, et al. Autologous chondrocyte implantation using a bilayer collagen membrane: a preliminary report. J Orthop Surg (Hong Kong) 2003;11(1):10–5.

54. Giannini S, Buda R, Vannini F, et al. Arthroscopic autologous chondrocyte implantation in osteochondral lesions of the talus: surgical technique and results. Am J Sports Med 2008;36(5):873–80.

55. Gillogly SD, Myers TH, Reinold MM. Treatment of full-thickness chondral defects in the knee with autologous chondrocyte implantation. J Orthop Sports Phys Ther 2006;36(10):751–64.

56. Peterson L, Brittberg M, Kiviranta I, et al. Autologous chondrocyte transplantation. Biomechanics and long-term durability. Am J Sports Med 2002;30(1): 2–12.

Treatment Algorithm for Osteochondritis Dissecans of the Knee

James L. Carey, MD, MPH[a],*, Nathan L. Grimm, BS[b]

KEYWORDS

- Osteochondritis dissecans • Knee • Sports medicine • Treatment • Algorithm

KEY POINTS

- Determining skeletal maturity as well as osteochondritis dissecans (OCD) lesion stability and salvageability are important to any OCD treatment algorithm.
- Given the paucity of high-quality studies of OCD treatment, algorithmic protocols are based on expert opinion, primarily.
- Future research in the management of OCD through high-quality studies will help elucidate the most effective and appropriate treatment management strategies for OCD.

BACKGROUND

The cause of osteochondritis dissecans (OCD) has been perplexing for more than 130 years. Since Konig's[1] early description of OCD, numerous hypotheses have abounded. These hypotheses include trauma,[2–6] genetics,[7–10] inflammatory causes,[11] and vascular abnormalities.[12,13] However, no single hypothesis has gained consensus agreement in the orthopedic community. Nonetheless, given the increased incidence of OCD in the athletic population, most in the sports medicine community agree that repetitive microtrauma plays at least some role in the cause of the development of an OCD lesion.

This popular theory of microtrauma gained support because the classic location of OCD of the knee is on the lateral aspect of the medial femoral condyle. As described by Fairbanks,[5] OCD lesions in this classic location are possibly caused by repetitive

There was no outside funding for this study.

Disclosures: The authors of this work have no disclosures.

[a] Penn Sports Medicine, Department of Orthopaedic Surgery, Penn Center for Advanced Cartilage Repair, Perelman School of Medicine, University of Pennsylvania, Weightman Hall, 235 South 33rd Street, Philadelphia, PA 19104, USA; [b] Department of Orthopaedic Surgery, Duke University Medical Center, Box 3956, Durham, NC 27710, USA

* Corresponding author. Penn Sports Medicine Center, 235 South 33rd Street, Weightman Hall, First Floor, Philadelphia, PA 19104.

E-mail address: james.carey@uphs.penn.edu

Clin Sports Med 33 (2014) 375–382

http://dx.doi.org/10.1016/j.csm.2014.01.002

impingement against the prominent tibial spine. This theory had gained support by Nambu and colleagues'[14] biomechanical study showing that vigorous exercise may produce trauma resulting in bone collapse of the medial femoral condyle. This theory does not account for OCD lesions developing outside this classic location of the knee in athletes.

Given the relatively low incidence of OCD of the knee,[15–17] historically, it has been difficult to perform high-quality, prospective, comparative studies to ascertain the best available treatment options for those suffering from OCD. Most of the available literature on treatment has been retrospective in nature or small case series. However, many techniques for managing OCD lesions have been described, and options for management differ depending on several variables, including status of the physis, location of the lesion, stability of the lesion, and salvageability of the lesion.

This article provides a detailed discussion of the treatment options available for OCD in the athlete and includes a proposed treatment algorithm based on the senior author's experience.

CLINICAL PRESENTATION AND PHYSICAL EXAMINATION

The presentation of OCD of the knee is variable. The variability of the signs and symptoms is caused by the stage of the lesion when they present. A stable lesion that remains in situ likely presents as nonspecific knee pain that is poorly localized by the patient, externally rotated gait pattern, and a possible effusion.[18] Comparatively, a lesion that has progressed to instability may become a loose body and present with mechanical symptoms, including a catching or locking sensation. Anecdotally, we believe these symptoms are exacerbated by increased physical activity.

The athlete may be observed to ambulate with minimal antalgia. The knee may have an effusion. There may be some point tenderness. For the classic lesion, point tenderness localizes to the distal aspect of the medial femoral condyle with the knee flexed to 90°.

IMAGING

The importance of imaging in diagnosing and characterizing OCD lesions is well established and the goals of such imaging should be to identify, characterize, and stage the lesion as well as to follow healing.[19] Initial imaging of the knee should begin with plain radiographs[20]: weight-bearing anteroposterior, lateral, sunrise (merchant), and weight-bearing tunnel views.[21,22] From the radiographic series, the lesion can be localized and measured, morphology described, and patency of the physes recorded.[19]

Magnetic resonance imaging (MRI) has become the preferred imaging modality for further assessing and characterizing OCD lesions of the knee.[19] There are a few classification systems to stage OCD lesions based on particular MRI findings.[23,24] These MRI findings include a distinct OCD fragment, high T2 signal intensity observed between the parent and progeny bone, disruption in the cartilage interface between the parent and progeny bone, and loose bodies.[23,24] The authors recommend MRI for characterization of all OCD lesions in the athletic population.

TREATMENT OPTIONS FOR OCD IN THE ATHLETE
Conservative Management

In 1985, Bernard Cahill makes a clear distinction between the successful outcomes of juvenile OCD (JOCD) and the adult form (AOCD) stating, "JOCD and [AOCD] are distinct conditions. The former has a much more favorable prognosis than the latter."[25] The current terminology favors the use of skeletally immature and skeletally mature over the terms JOCD and AOCD, respectively. In 1989, Cahill and colleagues[26] reported that approximately half of patients with skeletally immature OCD of the knee in the athletic population go on to heal using conservative management. Others have reported greater rates of healing (81%) in similar athletic populations treated conservatively.[27]

In skeletally immature athletes with symptomatic yet stable OCD lesions, the senior author's preferred treatment is nonoperative. Specifically, the in-season athlete may wear an unloader brace to minimize weight bearing through the involved compartment of the knee. Otherwise, a cylinder cast can be applied for 6 weeks to minimize loading and shearing of the OCD lesion. Either way, it is important to communicate to the athlete and family that the key for these treatments is to eliminate pain. If pain is not eliminated, then the OCD lesion does not heal. Healing can subsequently be assessed on radiographs and MRI.

Despite the success of nonoperative management seen in the juvenile population, similar results are not echoed in the adult population. Skeletally mature OCD is believed to be simply a persistent skeletally immature lesion that has remained into adulthood.[28–30] Several studies have shown poor results of treating AOCD without surgical intervention.[28,31,32] In skeletally mature athletes with symptomatic yet stable OCD lesions, the senior author's preferred treatment is operative, because these lesions have little capacity for healing with nonoperative treatment. However, using an unloader brace to minimize weight bearing through the involved compartment of the knee is an option that may allow the athlete to compete for the remainder of the season. Of course, the following return-to-play criteria[33] must be met:

1. Ability to meaningfully contribute to the team
2. No catching (motion of knee is temporarily inhibited) or locking (motion of the knee is halted) sensations
3. Full range of motion
4. Normal strength
5. No effusion or trace effusion

Surgical Management of OCD in the Athlete

Many options are available for the surgical treatment of OCD lesions. For unstable yet salvageable OCD lesions, the senior author's preferred treatment is fixation with bone grafting (**Fig. 1**). Through an arthrotomy, the OCD lesion is carefully prepared by removing sclerotic and necrotic bone as well as fibrous tissue interposed between

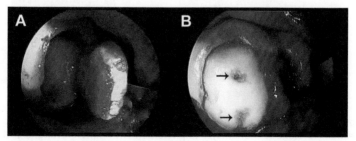

Fig. 1. Fixation and bone grafting of an unstable yet salvageable OCD lesion in a collegiate varsity football player. (*A*) Lesion hinged open. (*B*) Lesion in situ, after fixation with 2 variable-pitch screws (*arrows*).

the parent bone and progeny fragment. Autogenous cancellous bone is harvested from the ipsilateral proximal tibia from a region about 25 mm distal to the anteromedial joint line. The periphery of the parent bone is drilled with a 1.8-mm drill to facilitate the efflux of marrow elements to augment healing. In the setting of adequate bone on the progeny fragment, fixation is achieved with a variable-pitch metallic screw, which does not require subsequent removal. In the setting of inadequate bone on the progeny fragment (ie, fragmented bone or bone <3 mm thick), fixation is achieved with 1.5-mm solid screws, which do require removal about 8 weeks postoperatively.

For unstable and unsalvageable OCD lesions, the senior author's preferred treatment is autologous chondrocyte implantation (ACI) with bone grafting from the ipsilateral tibia (sandwich technique).[34] The key is to build the house on a satisfactory foundation (Fig. 2). Specifically, the OCD lesion is meticulously prepared to remove all sclerotic-appearing and necrotic-appearing bone as well as all fibrous tissue

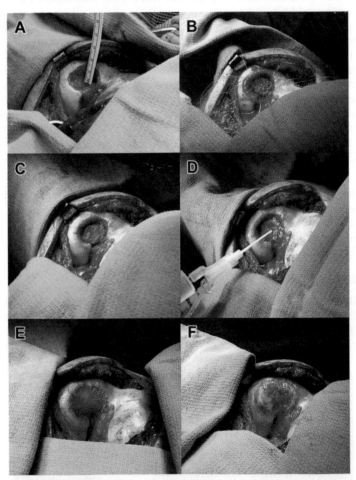

Fig. 2. Showing stepwise fixation of unstable and unsalvageable OCD lesion in a collegiate varsity wrestler. Autologous chondrocyte implantation with bone grafting. (A) Measuring depth. (B) After placement of autogenous bone graft and anchors. (C) Deep collagen membrane secured in place. (D) Application of fibrin sealant. (E) Superficial collagen membrane sewn in place. (F) Fibrin sealant applied to margins of superficial membrane.

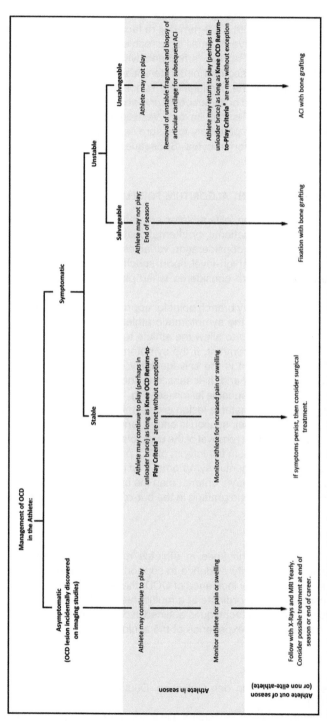

Fig. 3. Treatment algorithm for OCD of the knee in an elite athlete (for the purpose of this algorithm, an elite athlete is defined as a varsity collegiate level or professional level). [a] Knee OCD return-to-play criteria: (1) ability to meaningfully contribute to team; (2) no catching (motion of knee is temporarily inhibited) or locking (motion of the knee is halted); (3) full range of motion; (4) normal strength; (5) no effusion or trace effusion. Return-to-play decision making is often complex and depends on specific facts and circumstances presented to the team physician.

from the deep and peripheral aspects. Autogenous cancellous bone is harvested from the ipsilateral proximal tibia from a region about 25 mm distal to the anteromedial joint line. The parent bone is drilled with a 1.8-mm drill to facilitate the efflux of marrow elements to augment healing. Several small absorbable anchors (Microfix anchors, DePuy Mitek, Raynham, MA, USA) are rethreaded with 5-0 Vicryl suture (Ethicon, Somerville, NJ, USA) and then secured circumferentially in the parent bone about 2 mm distal to the interface of the cartilage and subchondral bone. The bone graft is placed under a porcine-derived collagen cover and secured in place with the suture in these anchors. Fibrin sealant (Tisseel, Baxter, Westlake Village, CA, USA) is placed deep to the membrane along the periphery to ensure separation of marrow elements and bleeding from implanted chondrocytes. Subsequently, ACI is performed in the usual manner.

AUTHORS' PREFERRED TREATMENT ALGORITHM FOR ELITE ATHLETES

For the purpose of this discussion, elite athletes are defined as those competing at a varsity collegiate, professional, national, or international level. In this athletic population, the surgeon must take into consideration variables such as timing with respect to the season, recovery time, and high-level, sport-specific demands. Issues like these are unique to the athlete and are considered when planning the most appropriate treatment (**Fig. 3**).

The stability of the lesion is a key branch point for appropriate management. As seen in our algorithm (see **Fig. 3**), in the symptomatic athlete, if the lesion is stable, the preferred treatment is to continue to allow the athlete to remain in sport if the criteria for return to play[33] are met. In contrast, if the symptomatic athlete has an unstable lesion, the next key branch point is the salvageability of this lesion. If salvageable, the athlete is removed from sport and their season is ended. We then proceed to fixation with bone grafting of the salvageable lesion (see **Fig. 1**), determining whether or not the lesion is salvageable. If the unstable lesion is determined to be unsalvageable, the athlete is removed from sport, their season is ended, and we immediately proceed to the first step of the ACI procedure: removal of the unstable fragment and biopsy of articular cartilage for subsequent ACI. In the interim of ACI preparation, the athlete may or may not experience an improvement in symptoms. If an improvement is observed and the athlete meets the return-to-play[33] criteria, then the athlete may continue to play in season and undergo ACI with bone grafting in the out-of-season period (see **Fig. 3**).

DISCUSSION

The management of OCD of the knee in athletes remains controversial, in part because of the lack of high-quality evidence to support one treatment over another. Moreover, given the relatively low incidence of OCD, these trials are difficult to power and logistically challenging to coordinate at a multicenter level. The treatment strategies and preferred management techniques outlined in our algorithm are based on the best available evidence and the experience of the senior author.

REFERENCES

1. Konig F. Uber freie Körper in den Gelenken. Deutsche Zeitschrift für Chirurgie 1887;27:90–109.
2. Conway FM. Osteochondritis dissecans. Description of the stages of the condition and its probable traumatic etiology. Am J Surg 1937;38(3):691–9.

3. Crawford DC, Safran MR. Osteochondritis dissecans of the knee. J Am Acad Orthop Surg 2006;14(2):90–100.
4. Detterline AJ, Goldstein JL, Rue JP, et al. Evaluation and treatment of osteochondritis dissecans lesions of the knee. J Knee Surg 2008;21(2):106–15.
5. Fairbanks H. Osteo-chondritis dissecans. Br J Surg 1933;21(81):67–82.
6. Smillie IS. Treatment of osteochondritis dissecans. J Bone Joint Surg Br 1957; 39(2):248–60.
7. Andrew TA, Spivey J, Lindebaum RH. Familial osteochondritis dissecans and dwarfism. Acta Orthop Scand 1981;52(5):519–23.
8. Kozlowski K, Middleton R. Familial osteochondritis dissecans: a dysplasia of articular cartilage? Skeletal Radiol 1985;13(3):207–10.
9. Phillips HO, Grubb SA. Familial multiple osteochondritis dissecans. Report of a kindred. J Bone Joint Surg Am 1985;67(1):155–6.
10. Stougaard J. Familial occurrence of osteochondritis dissecans. J Bone Joint Surg Br 1964;46:542–3.
11. Schenck RC Jr, Goodnight JM. Osteochondritis dissecans. J Bone Joint Surg Am 1996;78(3):439–56.
12. Campbell CJ, Ranawat CS. Osteochondritis dissecans: the question of etiology. J Trauma 1966;6(2):201–21.
13. Linden B, Telhag H. Osteochondritis dissecans. A histologic and autoradiographic study in man. Acta Orthop Scand 1977;48(6):682–6.
14. Nambu T, Gasser B, Schneider E, et al. Deformation of the distal femur: a contribution towards the pathogenesis of osteochondrosis dissecans in the knee joint. J Biomech 1991;24(6):421–33.
15. Linden B. The incidence of osteochondritis dissecans in the condyles of the femur. Acta Orthop Scand 1976;47(6):664–7.
16. Kessler JI, Hooman N, Shea KG, et al. The demographics and epidemiology of osteochondritis dissecans of the knee in children and adolescents. Am J Sports Med 2013. [Epub ahead of print].
17. Bradley J, Dandy DJ. Osteochondritis dissecans and other lesions of the femoral condyles. J Bone Joint Surg Br 1989;71(3):518–22.
18. Wilson JN. A diagnostic sign in osteochondritis dissecans of the knee. J Bone Joint Surg Am 1967;49(3):477–80.
19. Phillips MD, Pomeranz SJ. Imaging of osteochondritis dissecans of the knee. Oper Tech Sports Med 2008;16(2):52–64.
20. Mesgarzadeh M, Sapega AA, Bonakdarpour A, et al. Osteochondritis dissecans: analysis of mechanical stability with radiography, scintigraphy, and MR imaging. Radiology 1987;165(3):775–80.
21. Harding WG 3rd. Diagnosis of ostechondritis dissecans of the femoral condyles: the value of the lateral x-ray view. Clin Orthop Relat Res 1977;(123):25–6.
22. Kocher MS, Czarnecki JJ, Andersen JS, et al. Internal fixation of juvenile osteochondritis dissecans lesions of the knee. Am J Sports Med 2007;35(5):712–8.
23. Bohndorf K. Osteochondritis (osteochondrosis) dissecans: a review and new MRI classification. Eur Radiol 1998;8(1):103–12.
24. Dipaola JD, Nelson DW, Colville MR. Characterizing osteochondral lesions by magnetic resonance imaging. Arthroscopy 1991;7(1):101–4.
25. Cahill B. Treatment of juvenile osteochondritis dissecans and osteochondritis dissecans of the knee. Clin Sports Med 1985;4(2):367–84.
26. Cahill BR, Phillips MR, Navarro R. The results of conservative management of juvenile osteochondritis dissecans using joint scintigraphy. A prospective study. Am J Sports Med 1989;17(5):601–5 [discussion: 605–6].

27. Yoshida S, Ikata T, Takai H, et al. Osteochondritis dissecans of the femoral condyle in the growth stage. Clin Orthop Relat Res 1998;(346):162–70.

28. Cahill BR. Osteochondritis dissecans of the knee: treatment of juvenile and adult forms. J Am Acad Orthop Surg 1995;3(4):237–47.

29. Flynn JM, Kocher MS, Ganley TJ. Osteochondritis dissecans of the knee. J Pediatr Orthop 2004;24(4):434–43.

30. Kocher MS, Tucker R, Ganley TJ, et al. Management of osteochondritis dissecans of the knee: current concepts review. Am J Sports Med 2006;34(7):1181–91.

31. DellaMaggiora R, Vaishnav S, Vangsness CT Jr. Osteochondritis dissecans of the adult knee. Oper Tech Sports Med 2008;16(2):65–9.

32. Linden B. Osteochondritis dissecans of the femoral condyles: a long-term follow-up study. J Bone Joint Surg Am 1977;59(6):769–76.

33. Herring SA, Kibler WB, Putukian M. The team physician and the return-to-play decision: a consensus statement–2012 update. Med Sci Sports Exerc 2012;44(12):2446–8.

34. Peterson L, Minas T, Brittberg M, et al. Treatment of osteochondritis dissecans of the knee with autologous chondrocyte transplantation: results at two to ten years. J Bone Joint Surg Am 2003;85(Suppl 2):17–24.

Index

Note: Page numbers of article titles are in **boldface** type.

Clin Sports Med 33 (2014) 383–387
http://dx.doi.org/10.1016/S0278-5919(14)00014-3
0278-5919/14/$ – see front matter © 2014 Elsevier Inc. All rights reserved.

sportsmed.theclinics.com

Moving?

Make sure your subscription moves with you!

To notify us of your new address, find your **Clinics Account Number** (located on your mailing label above your name), and contact customer service at:

Email: **journalscustomerservice-usa@elsevier.com**

800-654-2452 (subscribers in the U.S. & Canada)
314-447-8871 (subscribers outside of the U.S. & Canada)

Fax number: **314-447-8029**

Elsevier Health Sciences Division
Subscription Customer Service
3251 Riverport Lane
Maryland Heights, MO 63043

Printed and bound by CPI Group (UK) Ltd, Croydon, CR0 4YY

22/10/2024

01777506-0001